MIGRAINE AND EPILEPSY

MIGRAINE AND EPILEPSY

JAN DE VRIES

From the BY APPOINTMENT ONLY series

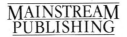
MAINSTREAM
PUBLISHING

First published in 1987 by
MAINSTREAM PUBLISHING CO. (EDINBURGH) LTD.
7 Albany Street
Edinburgh EH1 3UG

ISBN 1 85158 100 6 (cloth)
ISBN 1 85158 099 9 (paper)

British Library Cataloguing in Publication Data
De Vries, Jan, 1943—
    Migraine and epilepsy.— (By appointment only).
    1. Migraine   2. Epilepsy
    I. Title II. Series
    616.8'53   RC372
    ISBN 1-85158-100-6
    ISBN 1-85158-099-9

Typeset in 10½/12 Palatino by EUSPB,
48 Pleasance, Edinburgh, EH8 9TJ.

Printed in Great Britain by Collins, Glasgow.

Contents

FOREWORD 7

1 HEADACHES 11

2 COMMON MIGRAINES 19

3 CLASSICAL MIGRAINES 30

4 ABDOMINAL MIGRAINES 37

5 MIGRAINOUS NEURALGIA (Facial Neuralgia) 44
OPHTHALMOPLEGIC MIGRAINE

6 HEMIPLEGIC OR CIRCULATORY MIGRAINES 52

7 HORMONAL AND MENSTRUAL MIGRAINES 56

8 PSYCHOSOMATIC MIGRAINES 62

9 MÉNIÈRE'S SYNDROME 71

10 TINNITUS 76

11 VERTIGO 80

12 CONVULSIONS 84

13 EPILEPSY 89

14 PRACTICAL ADVICE 104

BIBLIOGRAPHY 114

Foreword

THE MAJORITY of illnesses can be helped by herbalism. Illnesses fall broadly into those which are self-limiting, because they tend to get better in time, without any help, chronic conditions which fluctuate but never seem to clear up entirely, as well as those caused by various types of stress. Only a small proportion (20%) of these are the result of an acute medical condition. It is this last category which may fail to benefit from herbal medicine, but even here many herbalists feel they can help if they can catch such serious conditions early.

I am not decrying the benefits of modern medicine. I would be the last one to refuse surgery for an ectopic pregnancy, but then all surgery is not necessarily of the life-saving variety. Much of it could be avoided by the intelligent use of preventative medicine, and it is here that herbalism proves so useful. A good herbalist is very much concerned with prevention. The problem is that most patients, in my experience, do not consult a herbalist until the damage has been done and very often as a last resort, having dragged themselves from one specialist to another, hoping for what increasingly becomes "a miracle cure", as their condition deteriorates.

FOREWORD

I know that Jan de Vries encounters this scenario as often as I do but I suspect he handles it with much more patience, humanity and foresight! This excellent book is one of a series he is writing which instructs the public about self-care. I am delighted that he is setting himself the task of capturing a lifetime's experience in words and passing on that treasure to other people. He has an extraordinary combination of in-depth knowledge and highly developed intuition and inventiveness. He displays more compassion and heart-felt concern than any other practitioner I have encountered. Above all, he is extremely practical. He would readily agree that although comfrey root poultices were used in the old days to mend fractures, an X-ray and a cast are preferable today. After all, a fracture may need to be surgically pinned. He knows more readily than I that acute appendicitis teetering on peritonitis calls for emergency surgery, not enemas and abdominal packs. But, like me, he sees a heart-breaking number of patients who, for example, have been on drugs for high blood pressure for ten or twenty years. This is surely not correcting or healing the condition. Such dependencies are the result of many years of ignoring or improperly treating the initial signs of high blood pressure or the malfunctioning organ system that induces the blood pressure to rise in the first place. If caught early, most cases of high blood pressure can certainly be cured without drugs. Time and again both of us see acute illnesses that have been badly handled and as a result they degenerate into chronic disease where drugs are then administered in an endless stream.

It seems today that antibiotics are prescribed like Smarties for the mildest bacterial infection and often for viral ones as well — where they are absolutely useless. There are some effective herbal antibiotics but where, rarely, allopathic antibiotics are required and their use justified by life-threatening illness, they would work superbly if the patient were not already antibiotic-resistant. This is the result of sipping away at too many antibiotic courses as well as eating hidden antibiotics in animal produce. It is Jan de Vries' great concern to teach his patients how to live and eat properly as well as helping them with appropriate herbal medicines.

The overall problem with a surgical or drug-based approach to illness is that it concentrates on symptoms as they arise, and therefore a patient is often at the furthest reach of the disease pattern before decisions as to how to treat it can be made. But most diseases begin years before such radical intervention is required. I am always somewhat bemused by patients who tell me they have just developed arthritis over the last six months. This is a classic example of a disease that takes years and years to build up in the body before manifesting its symptoms of pain, stiffness and swelling. Various types of headaches are endured for years and the painful symptoms vainly suppressed with allopathic medication. More than anyone else I know, Jan de Vries appreciates that by ignoring or suppressing such symptoms as they manifest themselves from babyhood or childhood on, we are pushing the body towards catastrophe. It is our experience that such catastrophe is hitting people at an earlier and earlier age. He tells me about treating diverticulitis in young children, being presented with juvenile diabetes in seven-year-olds and polyarthritis in teenagers.

While working punishingly long hours in unswerving dedication to his thousands of patients, he can still see through this gloom some light at the end of the tunnel. He is utterly convinced about the intelligence, love and humanity that shines in everyone and it is this conviction which shows itself so clearly in his writing and in his work. He is by no means a "back to nature" fanatic nor does he regard herbalism as a universal panacea. I suspect in an ideal world he would prefer to encourage the mingling of the knowledge and talents of the synthesist and the naturalist so that we could all benefit from the larger view without missing out on minute truths. I know he would like to see preventive health-care as embedded in herbal medicine employed to its best advantage so that it could enjoy at least an equal footing with modern interventionist medicine.

FOREWORD

This excellent and comprehensive book covers everything concerned with head pain and points out how vital correct diagnosis is. It discusses everything from common migraines through to epilepsy and, as with all his work, Jan offers practical and sensible advice. But there is a thread of God-given intuition that runs through everything he does and it is this that makes this book so illuminating. Read it, enjoy it and, above all, benefit from it.

Kitty Campion, MA, MH, PhD, RIr.

1

Headaches

"THANK GOODNESS for headaches," I once heard an elderly homoeopathic doctor exclaim. Because I was young and inexperienced, I considered this a very strange statement and could not help wondering how I was supposed to interpret it. He then continued to explain that headaches should be considered as an alarm signal, a warning that there is something wrong somewhere in the body. Headaches, therefore, should not be casually treated by merely taking an aspirin or a painkiller, for example.

A good doctor should investigate what the possible cause of the headache might be. In homoeopathy we do not aim to treat the symptoms, but the body as a whole. A seemingly simple headache may give us a clue to an often much bigger problem. Knowledge of this doctrine will give us a greater degree of insight and understanding of the statement by this experienced homoeopathic practitioner.

Dr Alfred Vogel explains the same doctrine in different words. During his lectures he will often tell his audience that when the church is on fire, the bells will be rung to warn everyone of the danger of the fire spreading. It is easy enough to stop the bells ringing, but the fire will spread relentlessly. This is only cured on the arrival of the fire engines to extinguish the fire.

This illustration contains the same message as the above-mentioned practitioner's statement about headaches. When subjected to a headache, one takes a couple of aspirins. By doing so, the ringing of the bells is stopped — the alarm signal is switched off. The fire, however, has not been extinguished, and may actually continue to spread.

Although it is often claimed to be "only a headache", especially if it occurs frequently, that headache may be the indication of something much more serious than just an inconvenient pain.

Although the main subjects dealt with in this book are migraines and epilepsy, I don't believe it is out of place if we first have a look at headaches. It is one thing to have an occasional headache, but quite a different matter to suffer frequent attacks of migraine. Mostly when people suffer headaches, these result from nervous tension. It is obviously more reassuring to think of one's headache as a result of nerves or a stressful situation. One should, however, not discount the possibility that it might be an indication of something more serious.

A variety of reasons could be the cause of headaches. The following are a few:

—a neck or back problem;
—sleeping in unaccustomed surroundings;
—an addiction to coffee or chocolate;
—even the price to be paid for certain indulgences the previous evening.

A headache may also point to hypoglycaemia, ie low blood sugar. Alternatively, it could indicate an allergy, hypertension, or even be due to a previous head injury. A disease from the eyes, nose, throat, ears or teeth could be to blame; or more seriously, it could be traced back to an intracranial tumour.

12

Fortunately the conditions mentioned in the previous paragraph relate to only a small percentage of headaches. Nevertheless, I still emphasise that headaches should never be neglected, especially if they are recurring ones. Let us not ignore the fact that a headache may be an alarm signal to forewarn us of possibly unsuspected and seemingly unconnected health problems.

I well remember the young lady who, on entering my consulting room, pleaded for some manipulation of her neck. It appeared that she frequently suffered bad headaches and she had convinced herself that they were the result of neck problems. Having listened to the background information with which she provided me, I tried to localise the pain. I had to tell her, however, that I considered it unwise to manipulate her without first being able to study some X-rays of the area in question. To be precise, I informed her that I would prefer it if she saw her own doctor for further investigation.

Fortunately I knew her doctor quite well and I made a point of telephoning him to talk about this patient. After he had examined her, he decided to send her immediately for X-rays and a brain scan. Within a short time a successful operation had taken place to remove a brain tumour and this saved her life. This goes to show how careful we must be in our work and again emphasises the fact that a simple headache may serve as a pointer to seemingly unrelated problems.

The majority of people who consult us, however, can be helped by some gentle manipulation or massage. If the cause of the headache is diagnosed correctly, much can be done to rectify the situation.

Unfortunately there is widespread misunderstanding concerning supposedly "simple" headaches. An elderly patient argued with me not so long ago that her chronic constipation had nothing to do with her headaches. Finally, I obtained her permission to treat her constipation and she did promise her co-operation, although she was by no means convinced of a possible connection. Both problems disappeared, however, as a result of the single treatment.

13

Why does this happen and, indeed, where lies the cause? Could stomach, liver, kidney or bowel problems really have any bearing on whether or not one suffers from headaches? I definitely believe this to be the case and it is for this reason that I dare to stress the danger of suppressing headaches with painkillers or other drugs.

A patient asked me recently if there was such a thing as a nervous headache. Of course there is: nervous headaches are a signal of an over-worked nervous system and patients who are prone to such conditions usually respond well to treatment.

"Why have my headaches disappeared?" asked another, youngish patient, after having followed a prescribed vitamin course. She could not understand the possibility of a connection between headaches and the recommended course of treatment. I then explained to her that, in her case, it was a deficiency of Vitamin B3 which had triggered off her headaches. When the level of Niacin had been corrected, her headaches disappeared.

Is it really as simple as that, or is there more to it? I strongly believe that every person's make-up is different and therefore individual diagnoses are required to get to the root of the problem. Once again I was reminded how difficult it could be when I was asked to treat a middle-aged lady who suffered almost constant headaches.

I had asked her if she had any idea why she should suffer these headaches and she insisted that she could not think of any possible reason. From her history I knew that she was badly congested with mucus and also that she regularly suffered from infected sinuses, but she refused to believe that she lacked oxygen. Yet she always looked pale and depressed.

More than anything else she needed to change her lifestyle to stimulate a more efficient oxygen supply. When I checked her over I also found that her liver was not working to capacity. As always with headaches or migraines, I will check the working of the liver, and I very often find that there is room for improvement here.

The liver is an important factor in the causes, and thus control, of headaches, migraines and epilepsy. The liver is the regulator of our health and acts as a very carefully tuned filter. It really could be compared with a laboratory and in that capacity, if taken care of, it is one of the most efficient examples of a refinery which nature has to offer us. Its greatest adversaries are some of the things we eat and drink, as this may affect the proper functioning of this organ and place it under stress. Among the results could be headaches and migraine.

However, we cannot then blame the liver, but rather ourselves. We tend to take our liver, this relatively small, but incredibly sophisticated organ, for granted. If only we could appreciate the fact that the liver filters 1,200 pints of blood during a period of twenty-four hours! Perhaps then we would recognise the marvellous achievements of which this organ is capable. Yet, on the contrary, we often overload the liver with alcohol, animal fats, nicotine, drugs and other unwise foodstuffs and fully expect this organ to process these in the normal manner. By doing so, we create a stress situation for the liver, making its task unnecessarily difficult.

So often, after patients have heeded my advice and followed a diet which has been especially designed to stimulate the actions of the liver, they will tell me afterwards how pleased they are with the results. The oxygen factor in these complaints is often forgotten, even though the liver thrives on oxygen.

Allergic headaches are mostly caused by eating the wrong foods or products, to which there could be an allergic reaction of which the patient is unaware. Again, the liver is given so much extra work that the alarm bells start to ring, warning us that help is needed. This help often consists of a change to a better diet, possibly some fasting, or the removal from the diet of those foods to which an allergy may have become apparent.

I remember one young man who constantly suffered headaches, yet for a long time he refused to accept that he was allergic to chocolate. Nevertheless, when he finally did overcome his choclate addiction, he felt so much better and his headaches disappeared.

There was also the patient whose headaches were caused by the atmosphere in which he worked. On top of that he had developed an allergy to dust. I treated him with homoeopathic remedies, together with a change in his diet, and he quickly regained his health and vigour. I still often meet him and he will always give me a wave and make a point of telling me that he no longer suffers those headaches.

Headaches which are due to sinusitis are also connected with what we eat and drink. The relatively simple step of removing milk, dairy products and salt from the diet, may result in the end of sinusitis headaches. I usually suggest that some honey is introduced into the diet of these people and they generally report afterwards that they feel so much better.

I feel very sorry for people who suffer headaches coupled with chronic insomnia, as this must be one of the most frustrating afflictions. They can actually lie awake for hours and hours at night. The cause here could be due to an infection, an inflammation or sometimes as a result of nervous irritability. Again to these people my advice would be that they take great care with their diet.

For the majority of these chronic headache sufferers I would suggest they follow the specific liver diet composed by Alfred Vogel. The main points of this liver diet are given below.

Recommended foods:
Lots of vegetables, especially taken raw
Salads dressed with Molkosan (a milk-whey product)
Buttermilk and low-fat yoghurt
Toasted wholemeal bread and rye crispbread
Sunflower or olive oil
Grapefruit, grapes and berries
Herbal teas
Apple and blackcurrant juice
Molkosan
Honey
Natural brown rice (see *Suggested preparation* below)

16

Forbidden foods:
Coffee, tea and vinegar
White sugar and white flour, as well as products prepared using these ingredients
Fruits which are not included in *Recommended foods*
Tinned products
Fried foods
Cucumber, cabbage, cauliflower or spinach
Spices
Sweets or chocolate

General recommendations:
Eat two plates of grated carrots daily.
Walk one to one-and-a-half hours every day.
Set one day a week aside for fasting. During that day only take apple juice, camomile tea and carrot juice.
Twice each day spend some fifteen minutes doing breathing exercises.

Suggested preparation for brown rice:
Place the required amount of rice in an ovenproof dish. Pour over boiling milk or water so that it reaches the level of one centimetre above the rice. Place the dish in an oven which has been preheated to its highest temperature. Cook for only 10-15 minutes and switch off the oven. Leave the rice in the oven for 5-6 hours.

Chop some vegetables such as parsley, chicory, celery and cress and mix these through the rice, with some garlic salt.

Reheat when required.

Many patients have benefited from this regime. I hear so often from patients, even if they have only followed this diet for a few weeks, that they are delighted with their reaction. We should always remember that when caring for our liver, it is in fact the whole of the body which is being cared for. No one can go wrong by following this diet. I especially recommend it, however, for those people who have suffered from chronic headaches related to either food allergies, incorrect dietary management, stress or tension. The liver is particularly sensitive to these influences and the diet will boost the correct functioning of this organ.

I cannot stress strongly enough the point that headaches are mostly symptomatic of more serious malfunctions. They must never be taken too lightly and one should always attempt to discover the cause of their occurrence.

When all possible influences have been considered, and the intermittent headache still persists, we may want to use some simple homoeopathic or herbal remedies. Another solution could be to apply an onion or horseradish poultice to the nape of the neck, the calves and the soles of the feet. There are plenty of other, equally effective remedies which can be used to overcome these unwanted and unpleasant headaches.

Among the several Vogel remedies I would reach for would certainly be included *Sanguinaria canadensis*. Nor would I hesitate to recommend Petadolor tablets, which are derived from butterbur (*Petasites officinalis*). I have seen many examples of the benefits obtained by patients using either of these remedies. Migraine Complex, by Vogel & Weber, is also excellent.

In the following chapters I intend to discuss some of the more serious forms of headaches and look into possible methods of treatment.

2

Common Migraines

AS BORNE OUT by my many patients there exists a large variety of migraine-type headaches. Many of these fall into the category of combined migraines, which can again be subdivided: a common migraine with classical symptoms, due to menstrual irregularities, or one in combination with abdominal problems. We will first deal with the common attacks, while also considering the complexity of symptoms.

Most medical handbooks teach us that the cause of a migraine is generally unknown, but there is evidence that it may be due to a merely functional disturbance. Cranial problems may also be at the root of it. Migraines can occur at any age, but again experience has shown that more women seem to endure them than men and that remission often does not take place till after the age of fifty.

Slight or severe headaches may occur after a period of depression, fatigue, restlessness, irritability or, sometimes, aggression. Some patients may be able to detect a pattern whereby they undergo daily attacks; while others will suffer once a week or even on a less frequent basis from a migraine attack. The length of an attack can also vary greatly, from a few hours for some people to several days for others. Some patients complain of nausea, others vomit or experience abdominal pains, while pains in the neck or contractions of muscles are also often mentioned as symptoms.

It is very important that a doctor or practitioner observes all the different symptoms of a migraine. Before he or she can come to a diagnosis it must be established what kind of migraine is occurring, because until that is known no effective treatment can be recommended.

Is it a common migraine, a classical migraine or perhaps a circulatory migraine? It could even be a "Sunday migraine". We know of so many migraines and their possible combinations but, as always, the most important task is to find out the cause for such an attack. Then a decision can be made on the necessary treatment, or whether it was an alarm signal indicating disturbances elsewhere in the body.

Only those people who have been subjected to migraine attacks themselves can fully appreciate the tremendous discomfort, inconvenience and pain migraine sufferers have to put up with. It is not unusual for a patient to complain of red objects dancing about in front of the eyes. Others try to describe the throbbing and banging sounds which they experience inside their heads or sometimes to one side of the head only. Many of them remark afterwards that, in their desperation, they wondered if it would ever come to an end.

Migraine always causes tension, not just during the actual attack, but also immediately prior to it as well as afterwards, when the person concerned feels drained. Both the body and the brain are involved and the whole mechanism seems to be the subject of an integration of tension.

Migraines are not a modern complaint, but have been with us for thousands of years. We know from Hippocrates, the father of medicine, that the ancient Greeks complained of headaches coupled with double vision. In old English medical literature we can read how medical people classified migraines, although they differed from us in their approach to the problem. Some held the view that only the intelligentsia suffered from migraines, and others maintained that victims of migraine attacks were to be found at every level of society.

Harold Wolff, an American neurologist and psychiatrist, discovered many years ago a certain instability of the arteries. The contraction of the large and small arteries caused by speeding up the heartbeat were, for him, an indication of what happened to a migraine patient. It was soon discovered that allergies and certain foods could bring on or exacerbate a migraine.

Cheese, wine, or meat extracts containing tyrosine are often the cause of a migraine. Chocolate and alcohol can also serve as unfavourable influences. There are, however, many more possible causes, which will be discussed in this book.

Fortunately, there are also many remedies, some of them extremely simple, which may be used to treat migraines successfully. Once again, every person needs to be treated individually. What works for one, does not necessarily have the same favourable effects for the next person.

The character of migraine pains can vary from throbbing, prickling, stretching, piercing or radiating pains to upward or downward pressure on specific areas of the head.

The common migraine is most often experienced as a violent throbbing pain in one of the temples; this intense pain can last for longer or shorter periods. Nausea or a feeling of sickness is frequently the result of a common migraine and when a sufferer manages to vomit, a feeling of relief is usually experienced afterwards.

What is often referred to as a blinding headache, or a blurring of vision, could be due to either nasal or abdominal problems.

A true migraine headache has diverse origins. During my studies in the Far East I learned that treatment of any migraine headache begins by treatment of the liver and gall bladder, and as it is very important with any migraine-type of headache that there is a regular bowel movement, this is checked as well. Hence the reason that dietary management is considered to be of such importance. The migraine sufferer who has emptied the stomach, or has good bowel movement, immediately feels a measure of relief. Prevention is always better than cure and therefore these important organs and functions deserve proper care. Never underestimate the sensitivity of the liver and the kidneys to emotion — tension, fear and stress should be avoided if at all possible.

Alcohol-induced hangovers could easily bring on a migraine headache. I well remember a highly placed officer who asked me to treat him for his frequent migraines. He usually felt well when he was at work, but on his home-coming he would relax with a bottle of whisky and a cigar. He did not realise that by his lifestyle he continued to push his liver into a stress condition. In his ignorance, he would encourage constipation by flopping into an easy chair after having spent his working day in a sitting position. As a result, most evenings at home would be spent in the grips of a migraine.

He had become quite desperate and therefore he fully co-operated by following the liver diet which I prescribed. He also agreed to cut down on smoking and his alcohol intake. His migraines subsequently started to diminish. He gained total relief after I gave him acupuncture, using gall-bladder and liver points. As the last part of his treatment I prescribed Boldocynara for him. This is a herbal remedy from the Vogel range and contains the following plants:

Cynara scolymus	— Artichoke
Carduus marianus	— St Mary's thistle
Polygonum aviculare	— Knotweed
Taraxacum officinalis	— Dandelion
Peumus Boldus	— Boldo
Berberis vulgaris	— Barberry
Raphanus sativus	— Radish
Mentha piperita	— Peppermint
Aloœ capensis	— Aloe
Lycopodium clavatum	— Club Moss

In the later stages of this patient's treatment I made some slight alterations to his regime and in the several letters of thanks I received from him, he informed me that he had become a different person altogether, now that he was free from the frequent attacks of migraine. He added that his wife was also very appreciative because he was no longer the morose person who endlessly lounged about in his chair.

Although I do not use acupuncture for every kind of migraine, if several symptoms occur in combination I might decide on this course of action. The flow of blood to the head is increased with acupuncture and this increased volume eases the pain during a headache.

Occasionally, I also teach these patients a few acupressure points and by following my directions they are able to relieve themselves of some of the pain during an attack. Mostly acupuncturists agree that during acupuncture treatment endorphins and encephalins — natural morphines — are released, the use of which is obviously infinitely better than that of a strong painkiller or other drug.

I must repeat here that prevention is always better than cure and when the first symptoms of a headache or a migraine become apparent, these acupressure points may be used to prevent it developing into a full-scale migraine.

I remember one patient who was beginning to develop a migraine pattern. She was still quite young and had positive views on medicine, showing a strong inclination towards naturopathy. She refused to use painkillers or drugs and felt that nature should run its course. I gave her dietary advice and performed some simple manipulation.

I then advised her to take hot footbaths while, at the same time, having an ice-cold towel wrapped round her head and neck. In her case that indeed cleared the problem and she was not troubled any more with headaches. There is often no need for complicated or difficult and costly treatment. It is more a matter of dealing with each case individually.

The big mistake is made when migraine sufferers take no action. Sometimes they adopt the attitude that, as they have this problem, they have to learn to live with it. We must not forget that these silent sufferers are the cause of more than half a million lost working days in Great Britain, at a cost to the Health Service of more than £3 million per annum.

I must agree with the general consensus that it is nearly impossible to find out how many people actually do suffer from migraines. I disagree, however, with the view there is no cure. No matter what type of migraine we are dealing with, once the correct diagnosis has been reached, ways can be found to alleviate the problem.

Migraines caused by tension, for example, are mainly rooted in the failure to relax. Some kind of relaxation is necessary to combat every type of migraine. Over the years I have come to learn that most migraine sufferers have a hard time learning to relax — to just sit back and let things happen, instead of winding themselves up about what is going on around them and worrying about how bad the situation may be. Learn to relax — put some effort into it, because it will pay off!

If we check the long list of likely causes of migraines it makes grave reading: nervous anxiety, emotional upsets, depression, traumatic shocks, excitement, plane and rail travel, bright lights, long periods of watching television, noise, sleeping tablets, alcohol, poor diet, hypertension, smoking . . . and so the list continues.

When I go over this, and there are actually many more influences I could add to it, I am reminded of a particular patient. He was a rough diamond of a man, with a broad Scottish accent, a heart of gold and with both feet on the ground. I had already noticed him in the waiting-room, banging his head occasionally, and when his turn finally came he told me his story.

He told me that he had been to see every kind of doctor under the sun, including a Harley Street specialist and a hypnotherapist. Finally, on the advice of his general practitioner, he had made an appointment to see me.

I listened carefully to his story, concerning his unbearable migraines experienced three or four times a week — a combination of common and abdominal migraines. His suffering was such that life, for his wife as well as for himself, was becoming unbearable. He had heard that I successfully used acupuncture treatment and wondered if he might be a suitable subject.

From the indications he had given me I concluded, however, that he was subject to common migraines and that it should not be too difficult to treat his condition. I decided that his diet needed some adjustment and I also gave him some remedies which I often prescribe for common migraines. One of the finest remedies I can think of is Loranthus (*Loranthus europaeus*) , derived from the mistletoe which grows on the wild oak. This is of great help for migraine and epilepsy as is Temoe Lawak (*Curcuma xanthorrhiza*), a not uncommon plant found in the Tropics.

He asked: "No acupuncture, no manipulation — only diet and these two remedies?" I assured him that if he followed my advice closely, his migraines would disappear and he left full of hope and enthusiasm. After two weeks he returned to see me, with the message that there had not been any change. I enquired whether he had followed my instructions and he said that he had. After another two weeks, there was still no change.

I began to fear that I had perhaps made the wrong diagnosis and again we went over his symptoms and the nature of his treatment. This time I also gave him some acupuncture treatment and manipulation. On his next visit — no change. He insisted on coming back yet again, but still there had been no change.

However, after having been in practice for a quarter of a century one becomes a bit of a detective and I asked his wife to come into the consulting-room. I asked for her co-operation and I went through the whole list with her. Then, finally, we came to the crux. He was a docker and he felt that after a hard day's work he was surely entitled to a double whisky. He was most surprised to hear that his daily treat could have any bearing on the lack of progress.

In fact that double whisky was the very mistake he had made and had invalidated the whole of the programme. I knew that his liver was under stress and I wondered why the liver diet had not produced more favourable results. His metabolic system was still under attack and therefore his migraines had not subsided.

Although he claimed it would break his heart, with a 'Scout's honour' he promised to do exactly what I had asked him to do for a period of three weeks. He came back to the clinic and announced: "This is absolute heaven — no more migraines for me." He told me that he felt a new man and promised faithfully to keep to the instructions.

At this stage I prescribed another remedy from the Vogel range for him, Centaurium, which is very useful for people who have slight stomach problems. It is also an excellent after-treatment for gall-bladder or liver problems. My patient happily set off for home full of good intentions.

Indeed, I met him again approximately twelve months later, when I was on a visit somewhere for a public lecture. He told me that it was absolutely unbelievable. He was a new man and did not know how to thank me. Of course, I was happy too, because I have treated many migraine patients — and who likes to admit defeat?

It was perhaps a year later that a lady with a slipped disc came into my consulting-room. I treated her for the condition and she looked happy and said to me: "You know, there were two people who recommended you. One was my boss, whom you have treated, and the other used to be one of our best customers. I am a barmaid and this customer suffered migraines for years until you treated him. He sings your praises whenever your name is mentioned. We had not seen him in the pub for a long time, but lately he has turned up again occasionally for a drink."

It cannot have been more than three months later that I saw my ex-migraine patient sitting in the waiting-room, banging his head again. This was the faithful customer of the pub where the lady with the slipped disc served behind the bar. I looked at him and told him immediately that I knew why he was back. I asked him: "Was the spirit willing but the flesh weak?"

He wondered if I possibly had second-sight and of this I could immediately reassure him. However, because of professional etiquette I could not tell him how I knew. The migraines were back though and, indeed, he confessed that he had again become a regular customer at his local. He had felt so well that he saw no danger in the occasional treat and, before he knew where he was, he had lapsed into his old habits again.

We had a good talk and he decided that he had no other option but to give up his regular tipple, because he now fully realised, although he enjoyed both a drink and the company, it was not worth the resulting migraines.

The advice I gave him goes for any migraine sufferer: please keep to the instructions from your practitioner and the migraine will usually disappear. Never give up hope, but use common sense: the instructions are given for your own good!

Unless a special liver diet is necessary, some more simple dietary advice will suffice for most migraine sufferers. The guidelines provided below should prove helpful.

Cut out:
Chocolate, cheese, citrus fruits and pork of any kind.

Cut down drastically:
Alcohol, nicotine and spices.

The more severe migraine sufferer needs a stricter diet, which is given below.

Breakfast:
Muesli served with prune juice.
Two or three slices of rye crispbread with blackcurrant or other jam made from berries.
Buttermilk or natural yoghurt.

BY APPOINTMENT ONLY

Lunch:
Choose from:
Salad using fresh, raw vegetables, except for peppers, onions, radish or watercress. Lettuce, celery, carrots and alfalfa seed sprouts are especially good in a salad.
Blended vegetable soup (including lentils, barley and herbs).
Potatoes, whole grains such as brown rice, barley or millet.
Two slices of rye crispbread or one slice of pumpernickel bread.
Toasted wholemeal bread.

Dinner:
Choose from:
Lamb — not more often than twice a week.
Beef — not more often than twice a week.
Fish such as haddock, plaice, sole, whiting or trout — not more often than twice a week.
Pulses such as soya beans, haricot beans, kidney beans, Tofu, lentils or chickpeas — at least two meals a week.
Brown rice and/or barley with sauté vegetables only — at least two main meals per week.
Potato or whole grains, brown rice and/or barley, millet and/or potato.
Fruits: choose from berries, pears or pineapple.

Beverages:
China or Earl Grey tea.
Herb teas of any kind.
Spring water.
Bambu coffee without milk or sugar.

Dressings, oils and condiments:
Dress salads with Molkosan, mixed with olive oil or cider vinegar.
Use plenty of herbs.
Use sea salt, Herbamare, Ruthmol or soya sauce.

Foods to avoid:
Chocolate, cheese, pork of any kind, red wine, coffee, alcoholic spirits, sweet foods, white sugar, cucumber, cabbage, cauliflower, grapefruit, lemon, oranges, banana, onions, yeast extracts, smoked or pickled foods, nuts, seeds, marmalade.

The above diet may be adapted to suit individuals, but it serves largely as a guide as to what is good for the migraine-prone person and what they should avoid.

I could also recommend that migraine sufferers take some extra vitamins — and most people benefit from some Kelpasan. These tablets contain pure sea algae and are rich in trace elements. Take one or two tablets first thing in the morning with some warm water.

3

Classical Migraines

"MOTHER, why do I always have a headache every time I have a day off?"

I can still hear my mother's reply: "Oh well, you are not the only person who suffers from Sunday migraines."

The expression 'Sunday migraines' was not at all unusual in the country of my birth, the Netherlands. Indeed, I came to recognise the symptoms myself. When I had been busy with my studies and holding down a part-time job in my spare time, often on Sundays at about mid-afternoon these dreaded headaches would start. Usually, I would have looked forward to a day of relaxation, satisfied that another busy week had passed — and then I would end up with one of these hated migraines.

Even when I was younger, the early signs had been present and although it may have been termed a classical migraine, it was not until much later that I realised what was at the root of it. I still thank God for the day that these migraines were cured because, although they had started out as more-or-less a 'Sunday migraine', they were constantly increasing in number as well as intensity.

At the end of World War II I had become a typical product of the war. As a result of the extreme shortage of food, my bowels had suffered, my kidneys had taken a beating and my whole metabolic system was in a mess. However, although I had been on the verge of dying, I was lucky and survived. As a result I was left with what at first were considered headaches, but which later developed into full-blown migraines.

I still clearly remember the day that a young Chinese practitioner looked at me and said: "Headaches — migraine — kidneys?" Despite his poor grasp of the language he managed to relate to me that my migraines were the result of the various health problems I had suffered in my youth. He applied acupuncture treatment and gave me some sound advice. In those days acupuncture was largely unknown in the West and I found it quite frightening initially. Since the two treatments at that time I have never suffered another migraine attack. Only occasionally do I still get a headache and I am the first to admit that this is usually self-induced; I will have overdone things, and the resulting stress sets the alarm bells ringing.

I do know, however, again from personal experience, that a classical migraine is much more intense than a common migraine and that it can last for quite a few hours. I also know that I used to pray for them to stop and I always felt sick during these attacks. I certainly remember that the intensity of these migraines adds up to something you would not wish on your worst enemy.

Classical migraines vary and the symptoms or, as they are sometimes collectively called, 'the aura' of the migraine, can cause rapid changes of mood. Sometimes memory or speech may be affected and even hallucinations can result. I remember well, that if an attack started during the night, I would consider that the worst possible luck, because then it would last for the best part of the following day.

I also remember experiencing cravings for certain foods. Certainly the foods I wanted would be the worst possible for me under those circumstances. Especially as a child, when I knew next to nothing about what was good or bad for me, I am sure that I must have unwittingly aggravated my condition.

This same problem appears when a classical migraine is influenced by hypoglycaemia — a low concentration of sugar in the blood. People who suffer from low blood sugar will find that when they eat a lot of carbohydrates, the problem will grow worse.

Not long ago I attended a special course on hypoglycaemia at the Basingstoke Clinic in southern England. It was a very worthwhile course and I certainly learned much about the dietary management of hypoglycaemia patients prone to migraines. It concluded that patients who have a tendency to migraines will often become nervous, irritable, dizzy, nauseated and anxious.

When the pancreas is over-active, sugar enters into the bloodstream. If this is not controlled by insulin, too much sugar will be removed from the bloodstream. If a large amount of sugar, or even honey, is eaten, over-compensation takes place and the vicious circle is established, the problems of which can lead to a migraine attack.

There are more hypoglycaemic patients who suffer regular migraine headaches than one might think, and a glucose tolerance test often reveals that here we find the true cause of the migraine.

Hypoglycaemia occurs mostly as a result of allergies to particular foods, although it can also be induced by the use of certain drugs, for example large doses of progesterone. The correct treatment is mainly found in the use of unrefined carbohydrates in limited quantities, as well as fats, and proteins which the body can break down into glucose. These will not produce such a high blood-sugar level that the pancreas is slowed down on its production of insulin.

My favourite remedy for use in combination with such treatment is Dr Vogel's Molkosan. Many of my patients who are hypoglycaemic or suffer migraines due to hypoglycaemic problems can vouch for this. Unless there are exceptional circumstances, I will advise them to take half a dessertspoon of Molkosan in a glass of water at breakfast, because the symptoms of hypoglycaemia or hypoglycaemic migraines mostly manifest themselves within a few hours of eating breakfast. It is certainly not impossible for a migraine to be triggered off by another meal, but it is more unusual. Breakfast seems to be the worst culprit. Emotional stress is also guilty.

The neurological aspects of these problems usually manifest themselves as either a severe migraine or headaches, accompanied by feelings of dizziness, numbness, blurred vision, blackouts, light sensitivity or, possibly, convulsions. Also noticeable could be a feeling of extreme fatigue, abdominal pains, backache, cold sweats, muscle and/or joint pain or even cramps.

Large meals should be avoided, as it is better to take six small meals a day rather than three big meals. In between meals eat some nuts, sunflower seeds, pumpkin seeds, sesame seeds or a piece of fruit. The main recommendations regarding diet for people who are subject to classical migraines due to hypoglycaemia are given below.

Foods to be avoided:
All refined and processed foods, white sugar, white flour, cakes, pastries, biscuits, ice-cream, white pasta, pies, puddings, sweet custard, white rice, marmalade and jams (unless sugar-free), chocolate, jelly, strong tea, coffee, alcohol, soft drinks, Ovaltine, hot chocolate, honey, salt (use Herbamare or Ruthmol), cereals containing sugar, chewing-gum, medications with caffeine, cough syrups, laxatives, ketchup, relish, sauces, mustard, Sorbitol, potatoes. Smoking should also be discouraged.

Limit the intake of full-fat cheese, grapes, plums, figs, bananas, prunes, raisins, dates, lentils, kidney beans, unsweetened fruit juices, bread and pasta. In addition, always be careful with your intake of salt.

Recommended foods:
Any vegetables and fruits which have not been mentioned

33

above. Peanut butter, unsalted nuts, whole grains, meat (except pork in any shape or form), eggs, milk, herbal teas, Bambu coffee, cottage cheese, yoghurt, acidophilus, soyabean products.

Often I have witnessed, with patients who arrived at the clinic round about mid-morning — in other words a few hours after breakfast — that while they were telling me their story a sudden change would come over them. I would realise immediately that I then was facing a patient in the grip of hypoglycaemic reactions.

A middle-aged gentleman came to see me who had been diagnosed as suffering from classical migraines. It often happened that while he was having a meal he would suffer these peculiar symptoms. It took me quite a while before I eventually discovered what was wrong with him. I was in the process of advising him on the use of typical remedies for such complaints, when I suddenly noticed while he was talking that a disalignment was apparent in his left jaw.

I decided that he needed jaw manipulation, which my dear friend, Dr Wilhelm Khoe, had taught me. It was almost unbelievable, but this patient later reported back to me that his headaches had become a thing of the past ever since the manipulation. I do agree that this may sound somewhat implausible, but the patient indeed has the last word and the results cannot be argued.

An eighteen-year-old girl told me about her symptoms, which again pointed to classical migraines. It did not add up, however, because the way she told me her story did not make much sense.

I went through the normal questionnaire with her:

—How long did her headaches last?
—Were they worse before, during or after the menstrual period?
—Was she constipated?
—Did she have indigestion problems?

—Did she have neck or back problems, or experience feelings of dizziness or blackouts?
—Did she suffer from cold hands and/or cold feet?

To each of these questions she answered negatively. She was, however, suffering so much that she had nearly reached the point of giving in and was wondering if there was any point in continuing life if this was what she would have to put up with all the time. She actually expressed a certain curiosity about death as she felt she could cope no longer. Although she did not give me the impression of being the suicidal type, she nevertheless spoke with some conviction. I searched my mind as to which treatment would be most suitable for her.

For anyone who does not believe in the power of homoeopathy let this case be a lesson. Here I had a case which was proving contradictory. In my mind I started to build up a picture of her physiological and psychological condition and on the strength of this I decided on the most suitable treatment. I gave her Natrium Muriaticum 30, and instructed her to take a dose of this remedy every two or three hours during an attack. After using this homoeopathic remedy during two attacks, she was free of her migraine and she has not suffered any further attack since.

If a classical migraine occurs as a result of abdominal problems, the patient is most likely to be a Nux Vomica type. A small amount of this homoeopathic medicine, given as a single treatment, is often all that is necessary to obtain relief.

Usually, with classical migraines, even minor dietary changes, such as eliminating citrus fruits, chocolate, cheese, spices, coffee and alcohol from the diet, as well as a reduction in the use of salt, can bring about a change for the better.

For the more severe cases my advice would always be to follow the specially designed liver diet, which I have already given in Chapter 1. Take three times a day ten drops of Loranthus, and also three times daily five drops of Boldocynara after meals.

In some cases also, it may be advisable to take Sanguinaria

and here again I would advise that this is taken in combination with Temoe Lawak. Both these remedies have already been mentioned in Chapter 1.

In the next chapter I will concentrate on abdominal migraines. I have already touched upon these, but they seem to be a more frequent complaint nowadays, especially with the younger generation.

4

Abdominal Migraines

A WORRIED MOTHER asked me the other day, in utter despair: "What in the world can be wrong with my daughter?" She had entered the consulting-room accompanied by a young girl of about fourteen years old, and the mother actually looked more disturbed at first sight than did her daughter. "We have been to so many doctors and have even been referred to a psychiatrist, because we were told that it was all in her mind, but the last doctor said that it could possibly be abdominal migraine — for what it was worth, because he was not sure about the treatment."

According to the mother, this had been a very strange statement, because as far as she was concerned migraine existed only in the head. She now wanted my opinion and wondered if there was indeed such a condition as an abdominal migraine. On that score at least I could reassure her. There definitely was a condition which we called abdominal migraine, and I would soon let her know if I agreed with that diagnosis.

I studied the young girl and we worked down the whole

list of questions, after which I was able to inform the mother that, in my opinion, the last doctor who had examined her daughter had been right. I had come to a few conclusions of my own while trying to make up my mind on the homoeopathic characteristics of this girl. I checked on one or two more things and was helped by the knowledge that I was dealing with a girl of above-average intelligence, with a quick-working brain and good common sense for her age. I knew that she was not malingering.

It may seem odd, but abdominal migraines do seem to be more prevalent among the younger generation. This could possibly be due to intense study or educational pressure, as parents often seem to be over-ambitious for their offspring and they are pushed hard to achieve good scholastic results. This condition is largely caused by stress, which can build up for various reasons.

This particular girl was extremely conscientious in her school work and that could well be the reason that she was affected by an abdominal migraine at times. Contrary to the mother's disbelief, this would definitely manifest itself as a severe headache. The abdominal pains and feelings of nausea, lasting for quite a while, would floor her totally and therefore interfere with her studies. This would upset her and make her uptight, which would start the cycle all over again. She seemed to be caught up in a vicious circle.

During a long chat with her I suggested several relaxation methods and referred her to my book on *Stress and Nervous Disorders* in which advice is given on exercises and other ways to relax.

However, for quick relief I prescribed Centaurium and Neuroforce. Both these remedies are available in the Vogel range of products. Centaurium is a fresh herb preparation containing *Centaurium umbellatum* (cornflower), and Neuroforce is composed of the following:

> Calcium gluconate
> Avena sativa

Glutamic acid
Lecithin
Natrium phosphoricum
Radix Ginseng

As I had hoped, she reacted very favourably to the treatment. Her mother made a point of keeping me up to date with her daughter's progress and later informed me that the headaches had totally disappeared.

Another case of abdominal migraine comes to mind, where the patient concerned was a seventeen-year-old boy. He too was very intense and suffered from tremendous intestinal cramps. The pains would sometimes drive him to screaming point, he told me. His doctor had diagnosed his condition as an abdominal migraine. The drugs which he was prescribed, however, had not proved effective; in fact they had actually aggravated the situation because he had turned morose and aggressive.

I felt for this young man because he was a sensitive person and I fully understood that he badly needed help. I set out by teaching him various ways to relax and I paid particular attention to muscle-relaxing exercises. One of his complaints was that he felt "heavy on the head" (his words) and I therefore suggested some special muscle techniques. These were basically intended to relax the head, and then that feeling would spread to total relaxation.

Using these techniques, together with a few homoeopathic remedies, the young man did very well and fortunately he once more became his former cheerful self.

When abdominal migraines occasionally appear after eating certain foods, we must always consider the possibility of an allergy. If you think that allergies are something confined to our present generation, you are mistaken. It is merely that this problem is receiving a lot more publicity than previously and also that, possibly because of our changing environment, indeed more people do seem to be developing allergies nowadays.

This went through my mind when I was asked to treat a young woman who complained of abdominal migraines, which would end in a severe headache which was difficult to shake off. When I listened to her carefully, I realised that these particular attacks usually appeared at a certain time during the morning. This immediately made me suspect an allergy. As a result of several allergy tests I did on her we discovered that she was allergic to wheat.

In order to first get a true picture of her condition, we decided, after having put our heads together, not to use any remedies for the time being. To test my theory I gave her a diet from which all wheat and wheat products were banned. She kept strictly to this wheat-free diet and at her next visit she told me that she had had no more migraine attacks. Better still, she told me that neither had she experienced any stomach cramps. Needless to say, she was delighted with the outcome, except that she was rather cross with herself for not taking action sooner and thoroughly regretted the time wasted.

Often in my books I have mentioned allergies, but this particular diagnosis was so quick and painless that I wondered again how many people could actually find relief from this problem if they took the bull by the horns and sought professional advice.

More and more people are discovering that they are allergic to something or other; but please do not suffer in silence — do something about it — find out what it is all about. I know that our knowledge can be compared with only the tip of a monumental iceberg and in my practice, over the years, I have seen this problem growing day by day.

The painless resolution of this young woman's problems intrigued me and out of curiosity I looked up some of my old study books. More than anything else, it was to check on how much I had been taught in my younger days about allergies as I was not sure how big this problem was seen to be in those days. I also wanted to find out how this problem was then dealt with. What I read rather surprised me.

One of the old study books I looked up was written by one

of the most eminent specialists on allergies, Dr Willem Kremer from Amsterdam. Back in 1939, Dr Kremer wrote a book on allergies and the treatment methods used. I must admit that even though I must have read the book at one time or another, I had forgotten how interesting the contents were.

Even at that time, Dr Kremer had realised that allergies were a growing problem, but I am sure that he would still have been shocked to see how quickly, and indeed how far, this problem has developed. I was impressed to read that he had already realised that the only way to combat this problem was by building up reserves of our immune system in order to stand the test of the many attacks on our health through the three energies we need for life, namely food, water and air.

In his book Dr Kremer mentioned the most common allergies, which displayed themselves as asthma, bronchitis, urticaria (hives), migraine, bowel problems and hay fever. I thought it interesting that he mentioned hay fever, because we now know that this allergy can be the cause of much more serious problems. The list of common allergies has grown tremendously with the passing of the years and the problems caused by them certainly give us plenty to think and worry about.

Migraine caused by a change in the blood circulation is due to a vaso-motor problem. Dr Kremer stated that caffeine and other food ingredients can cause sudden and dramatic changes in the circulatory system and this points to dietary control. It was interesting how in those days tranquillisers were normally prescribed for the relief of migraines.

Dr Kremer also used certain allergens and, in co-operation with a then well-known professor, he developed a de-sensitising method which provided the allergic patient with certain immune ingredients. With migraine patients, therefore, he set out to restore the balance of the blood circulation with the help of several remedies then available.

Since then, I have read much more on allergies as new publications appear frequently on this ever-growing problem. The one thing every specialist agrees on, however, is that practically any food product can trigger off allergic effects. It is not necessarily the food substitutes, colourings or additives which can be blamed; one can simply be allergic to a particular *item* of food. This was the case with the girl who showed immediate skin eruptions as a result of an allergy to fish. Even the smell of fish would trigger allergic reactions.

There was also another particular case which aroused my interest, where the person concerned was found to be allergic to lecithin, a fatty compound found in nerve tissue, blood, egg yolk and certain vegetables. This is most unusual, because it is generally considered that lecithin, a phospholipid, works medicinally for many people. In fact it is frequently used in the preparation of certain medicines.

Atmospheric influences can also have a bearing on the resistance of people to allergies. I have noticed, for instance, that people who were allergic to certain foods would suffer either abdominal or common migraines, but when using these foods under different atmospheric circumstances they would not display any symptoms.

In the 1930s the Amsterdam Clinic for Allergic Diseases developed specially designed rooms which were atmospherically protected from outside influences and maintained a constant climatic atmosphere. If an abdominal migraine patient is diagnosed as suffering from allergic reactions, desensitisation is one way to control the problem.

The reason why I have expanded on the subject of allergies is that I believe there to be a strong connection. So often, in cases of an abdominal migraine in conjunction with a common migraine, an underlying allergic influence can be traced.

Why are there so many allergic disorders, so many more than when Dr Kremer wrote his book? The answer to that question can be partly found in our knowledge of nutritional deficiencies. Chemical influences on food may be to blame for certain intestinal conditions such as *Candida albicans* and other chronic thrush problems. Also one must not forget that there is currently a general lack of variety in the diet and, all too often, convenience foods will cause a reaction.

I remember a middle-aged lady who had suffered migraines several times a week for years. She had never considered the possibility, but it was her habit of drinking a pint of milk daily which triggered off these migraines. By eliminating milk, without any further treatment, her migraines were gone within two weeks. From a letter she wrote I quote: "Oh, what freedom to be rid of these dreaded migraines! But to think that they were caused by cow's milk, which I drank because it was supposed to be good for me!"

A single allergy can be the cause of years of misery and let us be grateful of the methods available nowadays. These methods are totally safe and reliable — and that is more than can be said for the many painkillers and tranquillisers available for migraine patients.

Although thousands of patients can testify that they have become completely well again by eliminating certain foods from their diet, one has to be very careful to make sure that migraine problems which may have resulted are completely cured. I personally prefer to play safe and I find that Harpagophytum is one of the finest remedies for patients with allergic reactions.

Certainly in cases of abdominal migraines, I often prescribe Centaurium, occasionally Oil of Evening Primrose and to finish the treatment Harpagophytum, a herbal remedy containing the Devil's Claw root.

One patient showed immediate allergic tendencies on passing a brewery on her way to the shops and she benefited greatly from Harpagophytum. She claimed that her shopping trips to Edinburgh had once more become something to look forward to.

5

Migrainous Neuralgia (Facial Neuralgia), Ophthalmoplegic Migraine

Migrainous Neuralgia
THIS CONDITION is known by a variety of names, to name but a few: histamine headache, cluster headache or sphenopalatine neuralgia. The symptoms of this particular kind of headache are distinctive and often display themselves as an acute pain at the temple, over the eye, behind the ear, nose or cheek. Other facial areas may also be affected. Patients generally claim that the pain they experience is overwhelming and the intensity is enough to drive them crazy.

Where the average migraine patient generally prefers to lie in a darkened room, people suffering from migrainous neuralgia mostly choose to sit upright and more often than not find themselves pacing up and down in utter frustration. I have even seen them literally banging their heads against the wall.

Fortunately, on the whole, the pain does not last too long — rarely more than a few hours — although it is so intense that the patients cannot possibly concentrate on ways to relax, as they are totally restless as a result of the pain.

During my many years in practice I have seen quite a number of patients with migrainous neuralgia, which has given me the chance to investigate some of the possible causes of this type of migraine. I have also learned that, as with any other migraine, this type too can point to more serious problems.

Some patients may have an attack of migrainous neuralgia at regular intervals, where others will only experience them once or twice a year. However, when a migrainous neuralgia does occur regularly, it must be investigated. I have noticed that after regular occurrence there may follow a period of remission, but it really is extremely important to find out what is at the bottom of it.

Although this migraine seems more common in men than in women, in both cases it is equally true that it serves as an indication or an alarm signal of more serious problems and at least in this respect both sexes are the same.

Many of the symptoms of migrainous neuralgia can be treated by the general diet for migraines. Very often, however, we have to resort to homoeopathic remedies, as a possible cause of migrainous neuralgia is the presence of a miasma. This is a symptom left over from a previous problem, such as an infection, inflammation or a virus, and the symptoms of such a migraine will probably indicate something more serious. If neglected, the possibility exists that the condition of a degenerative illness is allowed to continue unhindered.

I remember a multiple sclerosis patient who came to the clinic for treatment. While I meticulously tried to piece together his case history, I discovered that he had initially suffered from cluster headaches. At first these had been diagnosed as pseudo migraines and later as normal migraines. However, when we discussed the various symptoms together, I soon found out that these had in fact been attacks of migrainous neuralgia. Unfortunately, he had not tried to obtain treatment at the time.

When at a later stage he was queried by a multiple sclerosis specialist about his early symptoms, it appeared that the

45

migraines had increased in frequency; meanwhile double vision, lack of bladder control and imbalance problems had slowly developed. Indeed I found a miasma of a previous viral infection and in my mind there was no doubt that here we had hit on the cause of the original migrainous neuralgia. Had this been treated properly at the time, he might never have become a serious multiple sclerosis patient, but unfortunately he had since totally lost his mobility.

I mention this case because I have a strong feeling that here we may be dealing with indications of more serious problems to come if the condition is allowed to continue unchecked. I have come across this pattern quite a few times and therefore I must stress that such migrainous neuralgia attacks always warrant thorough investigation. Whatever the original infection, inflammation or virus may have been, when severe attacks of migraine occur, we must not neglect them.

I once attended a very interesting lecture given by Father Wilhelm, as he is known in the United States. In his lecture he only briefly touched on the point of degenerative disease, as the lecture mainly centred on his long years of research into different viruses.

We also hear of migrainous-type headaches among the symptoms of rheumatic fever. The American, Dr Edward Rosenow, has undertaken research in the field of viral infections for over sixty years. He has written 450 medical papers since 1925, mainly on how different viruses can affect the human body. Father Wilhelm mentioned in his lecture that he had exchanged notes with Dr Rosenow on several occasions and they also discussed the streptococcus bacteria. When Dr Rosenow stated, in 1925, that the streptococcus bacteria could possibly be linked with rheumatic fever, the medical world in general laughed at him. However, twenty-five years later they had to agree that he had been right.

Dr Rosenow said that billions of organisms exist in the human body. He claimed that a specific streptococcus bacteria was thought to be responsible for certain diseases and he had developed a special technique which enabled him to multiply this virus millions of times. He also discovered the strength of the streptococcus bacteria and stated that it took ninety hours of boiling in H_2O_2 (hydrogen peroxide) to destroy this bacteria. The streptococcus bacteria, for example, is so strong that it can maintain life in temperatures ranging from 350° above zero to 150° below zero. He also found that it is so small that a trillion of this virus can live in one square centimetre, alongside other bacteria. Both of these facts go to show what formidable opposition we are up against.

Dr Rosenow found that if he injected the patient with the destroyed streptococcus bacteria, this served successfully as an antibody.

During neurotropic tests he discovered that this bacteria could also be responsible for those cases where people were mentally affected. Moreover, he claimed that certain types of cancer could have been caused by a virus infection. Although the medical world kept him at arm's length and refused to subscribe to his theories, he certainly has found ways in which these particular problems may be treated and I personally do feel that H_2O_2 may be beneficial in certain cases. However, it is best used under strict medical guidance.

It has amazed me in the past few years how many old methods of treatment have once again become commonly used. I remember so well that my grandmother prescribed H_2O_2 for people with throat problems. She always maintained that many illnesses could start with a sore throat or pharyngitis, and that the best thing to treat this would be to use 3 per cent hydrogen peroxide, diluted in a cup of water and used to gargle. If some of the solution was accidentally swallowed, it would do no harm.

Even today it is recognised that the use of hydrogen peroxide can be of the greatest help in some serious illnesses. In very small doses it is harmless, although with more serious problems it is obviously better to have this prescribed under medical supervision.

However, for all migraine types as well as for the tinnitus patient it can be a tremendous help. First thing in the morning and very last thing at night five drops of hydrogen peroxide (30%) should be taken in a full glass of water. This can be increased to ten drops in a full glass of water after a few weeks. Let me stress again, however, the importance of patients keeping strictly to that amount; any increase should only be decided by qualified medical practitioners.

Many patients have found great benefit from this remedy and, of course, the extra oxygen input has shown some remarkable results in more serious diseases.

To me, migraines serve as a warning because of a possible link to one or more of the many viruses already known to us. Homoeopathic antidote therapies may supply us with the correct answer here.

This reminds me of a young woman who is employed in one of the local banks. Whatever she had picked up I still do not know for certain, but she suffered severely from facial neuralgia and migraine headaches. I successfully treated her with high doses of Oil of Evening Primrose capsules — in which the extract of the Evening Primrose is combined with a fish oil — and also prescribed Vogel's Harpagophytum drops. By the time she came to me for treatment, she had already become aware of difficulties in her balance and tingling sensations in her fingers, and she also experienced slight bladder control problems. We were both equally delighted with the success of her treatment.

I therefore dare to say it again: when inexplicable migraines or headaches occur on a more or less frequent basis, please do go and have it seen to. By doing so, irreversible health damage may be prevented or avoided by taking the appropriate, and timely, action.

Ophthalmoplegic Migraine
Ophthalmoplegic migraine is fortunately a rare kind of migraine. It can seriously affect eyesight due to restriction of the movement of the muscles of the eye. Although we do not come across this particular type of migraine often, whenever I do have a suspected case of ophthalmoplegic migraine, I will

not attempt treatment until I have had a chance to study X-rays of the patient. Mostly, however, I will refer such a patient to a neurologist, as we might encounter an aneurysm or other neurological problems.

If, however, it is a straightforward case of ophthalmoplegic migraine, when often a temporary swelling in the eye may be observed, I might use acupuncture or cranial osteopathy treatment.

I came across a very interesting case of a girl whose pupil of the left eye was slightly bulging in comparison to the right one. Immediately upon seeing her, I referred her to a neurologist. The specialist saw that all the necessary tests were taken, but no signs were found that there was anything seriously wrong with her. When she experienced a migraine attack the eye would swell slightly, not leaving us in any doubt about an oedema. Yet, after the attack she would be all right. This had been occurring for quite a number of years and as all the tests were clear and the diagnosis was positive in that there was nothing seriously wrong, I treated this girl successfully with acupuncture.

I combined the acupuncture treatment with some homoeopathic preparations:

—Loranthus, which I have already mentioned;
—Venalot, a capsule to promote circulation;
—Hyperisan, to strengthen the veins.

Hyperisan is composed of:

Achillea millefolium	— Yarrow
Aesculus hippocastanum	— Horse chestnut
Hypericum perforatum	— St John's Wort
Arnica montana e radix	— Arnica herb and root

When this patient arrived for her second appointment she told me that she had been very much worse after her first acupuncture treatment. This, unfortunately, is sometimes the case with acupuncture and occasionally people are frightened sufficiently to make them decide to discontinue the treatment.

I had, however, forewarned her of this possibility and she remained willing to co-operate. Thank goodness that after her second treatment she started to feel a bit better. After two treatments she claimed to be right as rain.

With these sorts of headache treatment can actually be rather tricky, as there could be a remission for a longer period of time, and then the pains could again rear their ugly heads. I had not seen her for a few years when I was consulted on a different matter by her mother. I was delighted to hear from her that her daughter had never experienced any further problems.

Ophthalmoplegic migraines could have various causes and we often have to seek their origin without the visible help in our diagnosis as had been the oedema in the young girl's eye.

I was once asked to treat a youngish man whom I suspected to be suffering from ophthalmoplegic migraine. I took a long time to come up with a possible cause and I finally fastened onto a very slightly dilated pupil, which could be a sign of dental amalgam poisoning. This patient underwent the Dr Voll's test and indeed I found confirmation of my tentative diagnosis.

There is some confusion and disbelief in the medical world on the subject of dental amalgam poisoning. I have found, however, as have quite a few of my colleagues, that such poisoning could well be accountable for such or similar problems.

When I urged this patient to have all his dental amalgam fillings removed and replaced by composite fillings, the ophthalmoplegic headaches indeed disappeared.

In one of my earlier books — on *Multiple Sclerosis* — I have written in detail of the possible dangers of dental amalgam fillings and with some of the more serious migraine cases it would be wise not to ignore this possibility. These fillings can definitely be the cause of excessive toxicity, influencing the total general health of the patient.

The treatment of ophthalmoplegic migraines may require cranial osteopathy, but sometimes I come across a case where

I consider jaw adjustment to be useful. I have already discussed the occasional need of jaw adjustment in a previous chapter and again for an ophthalmoplegic migraine this treatment may be called for.

In the United States the term "jawlash" is frequently used, whereas in Britain we are only familiar with the term "whiplash". The basic principle is the same, only it relates to a different part of the skeleton. Problems such as pains in the head, facial pains, balance difficulties, blurred vision, altered sensitivities, tingling in the arms and fingers could all be due to jawlash. Although it may sound improbable, a jawlash adjustment can indeed prove to be the ideal method to overcome such problems.

Whenever I use this method of treatment, I combine it with Vitamin B complex and an anti-inflammatory herbal preparation for which I mostly choose Dr Vogel's Echinaforce. Usually this will take care of the disorder, but if there has been an injury of any kind I may also prescribe Arnica.

The two serious migraines we have dealt with in this chapter need careful study before a suitable method of treatment can be decided on.

I can report, however, that in most cases where I have been consulted by patients with a lengthy history of headaches, and where other treatments have failed to produce the required results, both migraines have responded well to H_2O_2 hydrogen peroxide treatment and to homoeopuncture. The latter is an acupuncture treatment where the needle has been dipped in a homoeopathic extract, in this instance, Belladonna. The dipped needle will then be placed in the required acupuncture point.

Sometimes laser treatment will also bring relief and if care is taken and the correct diagnosis has been reached, these headaches may be cured.

6

Hemiplegic or Circulatory Migraine

ALTHOUGH HEMIPLEGIC MIGRAINE has always been considered to fall into the category of rare migraines, and rightfully so, I have noticed a recent increase in this type.

Hemiplegic migraine attacks can last for anything from several hours to a few days, and, although unusual, they can even last for a whole week. The pain is excruciating and I do feel sorry for the people who are thus inflicted, because if they had taken better care of their general circulation, they might not now be suffering so much. Again, as previously pointed out, an attack of hemiplegic migraine should be considered as an alarm bell: there is something wrong somewhere in the body, and in this case it is frequently the circulation.

I have never failed to be surprised when investigating this kind of migraine. Many migraine patients suffer cold hands and feet, but these patients seem to suffer excessively from such symptoms. Exercises to improve the circulation can sometimes actually trigger an attack.

I remember a mother of two young children who consulted me. She had been to several orthodox doctors and to colleagues of mine in alternative medicine and finally ended up at our clinic. I realised that she had already explored all the available channels of help and there was no doubt in my mind that she primarily needed treatment for circulation problems.

The treatment I prescribed for her luckily produced a gradual improvement in her circulatory system. Although she had previously been prescribed a variety of remedies, whether homoeopathic, herbal or otherwise, there had been absolutely no change in her condition.

First of all I suggested manipulation, as I believed her migraines to be due to a restricted blood supply to the brain. As the free transport of blood was blocked, I adjusted the third cervical vertebra and she immediately informed me anxiously that she felt dizzy. I advised her not to move, and to take things easy; after a while she said that she felt better and I was able to tell her that, due to the manipulation, the restriction in the blood circulation had been removed. She told me that she had always been scared at the thought of manipulation — and justifiably so. She had heard of people whose condition had actually deteriorated after a manipulation. Neck or cranial manipulation must *always* be undertaken with the greatest care and only ever by experienced practitioners.

After she had sat down for a while she felt a certain freedom and claimed that her head seemed to feel lighter. I insisted that she stay for a while longer till the situation had normalised itself and in the meantime gave her some further advice as to how to improve her blood circulation in general. I also prescribed Hyperisan for her, together with Venalot. This is a herbal remedy I obtain from Germany and it contains extracts of Melilot stand sicc. and rutin.

Venalot is a marvellous remedy for stimulating ailing circulation and does not inhibit blood coagulation. This patient progressed very well and, as I also treat her children, I still see her occasionally. Over the latter years she has not been bothered again by any headaches, for which she is extremely grateful.

Another patient with similar problems was a very studious

young man. Initially I blamed an excessive anxiety to perform well in his university studies, but after thorough investigation I realised that he needed treatment as a hemiplegic migraine patient. As he had not had any success with previous treatment, he showed his desperation when he said: "Please do whatever you think necessary."

I knew that he was very busy, but he agreed to a programme I worked out for him. The treatment programme for this patient included the general diet for migraine sufferers and the homoeopathic remedies Loranthus and Hyperisan.

I also instructed him on what we at the clinic refer to as 'the cold dip'. This is a form of hydrotherapy, intended to influence and stimulate the circulation and therefore ideally suited for those people who suffer from cold hands and feet.

The following routine should be followed each morning on rising and each night before retiring. Place a basin of cold water at the side of the bed with a towel at the ready. When getting up in the morning, place both feet into the water. After having counted to ten, move the feet onto the towel and dry them. Exercise the toes as if trying to pick up a marble for anything from ten to thirty times.

On retiring, repeat the morning procedure and you will find that your feet are as warm as toast when you get into bed. The importance of this exercise is that it should be done for a minimum of sixty days if you want to feel the full benefit. This exercise may look simple, and indeed does not involve any financial outlay, only willpower and perseverance. If carried out as stated, it will definitely have a remedial effect.

After three to four weeks this particular patient reported that he had made considerable progress and expressed his whole-hearted gratitude for the advice, which indeed he had followed strictly. He became a much less intense person and felt that he was performing better in his studies, which he considered a valuable bonus.

Hemiplegic migraine is no different to the other types of migraines mentioned, in that it requires careful monitoring. The attitude of the patient can make all the difference to the progress attained; co-operation and the use of common sense are both vital. I understand that the spirit is often willing, but that the flesh is weak, but by following advice the reward will often be a return to good health, unless there is something seriously wrong. Mostly, the attitude of the patient is the deciding factor in his or her recovery.

7

Hormonal and Menstrual Migraines

DEPENDING ON THEIR AGE, I will ask female migraine patients on their first visit to the clinic: "Is your migraine worse before, during or after menstruation?"

It is important that I obtain an answer to this question while I still have an open mind regarding the final diagnosis. The answers obviously differ, but they could be the first pointer to a hormonal type of migraine. It would not be the first time that these migraines are wrongly diagnosed, and sometimes they are brushed off casually as a migraine due to hysteria. It is, however, quite possible that the migraine is drug related, for example when the patient is undergoing long-term oestrogen supplementary treatment. If the patient has been prescribed a course of hormone treatment and headaches subsequently occur, then one should not overlook the possibility that the hormone by-products could be the cause.

I have seen this happen with several of my patients. Many of us have heard of friends or acquaintances who had to discontinue the use of the birth-control pill, because it disagreed with them. Often this was indicated by migraines.

To be fair, I must immediately add that I have also treated ladies whose migraines were cured by hormonal administration.

If, however, the cause of the migraines points to hormonal interference and I consider it necessary to discontinue the hormonal treatment, I do this in conjunction with the doctor or specialist who had initially prescribed the hormone replacement course. A homoeopathic or herbal substitute may then be prescribed to take its place. If it has become clear that the birth-control pill is to blame, other methods of contraception will have to be found to ensure that these migraine attacks will not become a pattern of life.

I remember a young married lady who was undergoing oestrogen treatment and suffered severe migraine attacks. I advised her to discuss these problems with her own specialist, and they did indeed manage to find a method of contraception which suited her equally well, but which excluded the side-effects of migraine attacks. This, of course, is not always achieved instantaneously and sometimes it is a matter of trial and error before the desired results are obtained and both patient and practitioner are happy with the solution.

One lady, the mother of two young children, consulted me with horror stories of migraines which almost drove her mad. At first I considered her case to be one of classical migraine, but I soon discovered that she was the victim of a hormone imbalance.

Her migraine attacks were so severe that the only way to help her was by administering acupuncture anaesthesia to temporarily alleviate her misery. When she felt an attack of migraine coming on, she made her husband drive her to the clinic, where she would beg me for her 'trip'. She would be totally incapable of doing anything at all during one of these attacks and would be sick and miserable, which was in fact not characteristic of her when she was feeling herself. At such times it would be difficult for me to recognise her as the person I had come to know.

It certainly took quite a while before, at long last, we found the answer to her problems. Fortunately she had total co-operation from her husband, but nevertheless her family life suffered. The programme to which she finally responded was as follows:

—the general diet for migraine patients;
—Loranthus;
—a special natural hormone preparation which I had made up in Germany;
—Remifemin;
—Coliacron injections.

Remifemin is a homoeopathic remedy which contains *Rhiz. cimicifugoe* (black snake root) and is designed for menstrual disorders. It works in support of hormone therapy, without any side effects.

Coliacron is an enzyme injection which removes any deficiency in the functioning of enzyme complexes. The vegetative neuro-hormonal centre in the mid-brain is one of the links between mind and body. Disturbances in the functioning of brain and organs and in the development of the functioning of the neuro-vegetative system are favourably affected and removed by the use of Coliacron. An organism which is distributed in one or more functions, due to physical or mental influences, will manifest the following improvements:

—restoration of energy production in the nervous tissue and other organs;
—restoration of impulse co-ordination;
—restoration of organ innervation, including the hormone-producing organs.

Enzyme therapy is also conducive to developing the immune system.

If ever I could speak of gratification on the successful outcome of treatment, it was with this lady. She had suffered for years and had willingly tried different kinds of treatment, but was near enough without hope for the future by the time she came to me. Yet she co-operated fully and the end result was a happy one. When I see her occasionally, her husband, who mostly accompanies her, usually states: "If anyone needs convincing that alternative treatment is effective, she is a prime example!"

Hormonal activity can be responsible for certain physiological and emotional changes in women. One of my Dutch lecturers was fond of reminding his students of our fractional knowledge relating to the endocrine system, and that we were still very much in the dark on what we should and should not do. It is crucial when treating menstrual migraines that we find out as much as we possibly can about the nature of the menstrual periods as well as the timing. Only when that has been established may successful treatment be decided.

One of the things I was taught during my training was that migraines belong in the classification of vascular headaches and that vascular contraction and/or dilation are a common feature.

Physiologically, the responsibility lies with our vegetative nervous system, in other words one half of our central nervous system. We have a large and varied input into our central nervous system, but it is the vegetative autonomous nervous system which controls the internal organs.

Our blood vessels, too, are controlled by the vegetative nervous system. If, however, the sympathetic part of the vegetative nervous system is out of alignment with the parasympathetic part, stress situations can occur, sometimes displaying themselves as migraine headaches.

The vegetative nervous system is complex and I do not want to dwell here on its range of functions. Nevertheless, questions arise about the behaviour pattern of the vegetative nervous system during a migraine attack. I will briefly mention the possible cause and consequence:

The vegetative nervous system is ruled by the hypothalamus, which is housed in our brain. There we find the central hormone gland — the pituitary gland — which is closely connected with the menstrual cycle. Hence a possible reason that through the contraction of the blood vessels during a menstrual cycle a migraine may occur. This indicates just how closely connected the pituitary gland is to the menstrual cycle and this could possibly explain why some women suffer menstrual migraines and others do not. It all depends on how well the gland functions.

Hormones produce ingredients which will enter the bloodstream and, under certain circumstances, will cause physiological changes. The function of the brain as the centre of our nervous system is responsive to the performance of the pituitary gland. Anatomically, the pituitary gland is in close contact with the emotional centre of the brain — the hypothalamus.

When the birth-control pill is introduced, the pituitary gland is given a break from its customary duties and its usual role in the natural functioning of the brain. Now we can recognise one of the reasons why we have to take such care when introducing hormonal products or substitutes. Sometimes Coliacron enzyme injections and Remifemin will meet the need and then further dependence on other hormonal products will be superfluous.

Remifemin — black snake root — can relieve various disorders and symptoms, whilst at the same time avoiding hormonal therapy when there is no endocrinological indication. If hormones *are* required, the action is not interfered with, but complemented. This remedy has been proved to be effective as long-term therapy in hormonal disturbances of women during climacteric periods and during menstruation. Depressive tendencies after total extirpation are favourably influenced and no side-effects have been noted.

As Remifemin also has an oestrogenous effect, it is administered for female hormonal disturbances during dysfunction of the ovaries, juvenile menstrual disturbances, nervous diseases and migraines.

Sometimes migraines may occur in women with a slightly negative attitude to sexual experiences. Such an attitude may influence the pituitary gland in not only a physical but also a mental way as this gland plays a co-operative role between the ovary and the uterus. Sometimes there could be a disharmony, when young women may suffer a migraine attack due to fear of the unknown or insufficient sexual knowledge.

These migraines could then be cured miraculously by pregnancy. Similarly, it can be expected that menstrual migraines will disappear after the menopause or after sterilisation.

Women who experience uncomfortable swellings in their legs, ankles or even eyelids, could well end up with a migraine history, because a lot of credence is given to the theory that fluid retention or an oedema can trigger a migraine. However, others maintain that this again is an acceptable hormonal symptom and I personally believe that, with some natural remedies, such oedema problems can be overcome and when this happens the resultant headaches will also disappear. In such cases I prescribe a natural diuretic and sometimes Convascillan, an extract of *Convallaria majalis* — lily of the valley.

Hahnemann, the founder of homoeopathy, has given us this definition:

> The highest and singular mission of a doctor is to restore a patient to a state of health in a mild and definite manner.

In this context homoeopathy certainly comes into its own.

When an accurate diagnosis has been reached and the correct diet is taken in combination with natural remedies and objective treatment, the practitioner will feel fulfilled on seeing his patient restored to a state of health where he or she is free from pain and able to enjoy life to the full.

8

Psychosomatic Migraine

I HAVE ALREADY pointed out how important it is that the correct diagnosis is made concerning which type of migraine the patient suffers from. This rule applies even more so to psychosomatic migraine. It is extremely easy to stick the wrong label on a psychosomatic migraine, as we are dealing here with physical symptoms caused by a psychological problem. Time, care, understanding, patience and trust are essential between patient and practitioner.

An understanding between the two people involved takes time to develop and therefore psychosomatic migraines are often wrongly diagnosed in the first instance. When, as would be the case, the patient does not see any improvement in his or her condition, whatever level of mutual trust *has* been developed, will be easily eroded. The patient might then continue to search for treatment elsewhere. The endless process will continue, because the next practitioner who is approached may also not hit the nail on the head first time round, unless he or she manages to gain the patient's confidence immediately.

There is no doubt, however, that once a psychosomatic migraine has been correctly diagnosed, it can be treated successfully.

When we encounter a psychosomatic or an emotional type of headache, we have to study and investigate homoeopathic-ally what type of patient we are dealing with. In order to reach the correct decision, the patient's personality, characteristics, background, life history and all other possibly relevant information should be gleaned from the patient.

I realise how fortunate I was at the beginning of my career to have been taught by the best in their field, to name but two, Dr Alfred Vogel and Dr Benthum-Oosterhuis. When taking my first steps in the field of natural medicine, if I was ever puzzled, I could always fall back on one of my teachers, most of whom had long years of experience. One of these lecturers/ practitioners taught me a lesson in the field of diagnosing which I have never forgotten.

This was related to a friend of our family, a lady for whom we had the highest regard; a very organised person, married to a headmaster and the mother of two teenage children. Besides running the family she was involved in a lot of voluntary work and was greatly sought after for her organisational talents as a committee member and a conscientious worker.

I asked this friend of mine, who besides being a lecturer also ran a practice, to do me a favour and see if he could help this lady in connection with her migraines. After having spent an hour with her, he asked me how well I knew this person. I told him that she had long been a friend of the family, had an apparently happy family life and that her children were doing well. I filled him in on some general background information, which was not an awful lot when I thought about it.

Then he told me something I have never forgotten and which at that time I could hardly believe. He said that he was sorry, but he had not found any signs of physical irregularity which might account for her migraines. According to him, her migraine attacks were psychosomatic — caused by sexual frustration. I could not help showing my disbelief, because not for one minute could I imagine that such a thing could be the cause of her migraines. In fact I felt so taken aback that I doubted if I had made the right decision in referring her to him.

Although I am ashamed to say it, I lost some of the high regard which I had always had for him. He explained that because of the medical code of practice he could not break her confidence, but had only informed me of his diagnosis as I had originally approached him about her.

I left this particular patient under his care, as he was the experienced practitioner and I was just starting. Also, the fact that she was a friend of the family and the age-gap between us would have complicated things, and I had to believe that I was leaving her in better hands. Nevertheless, it was only human that my interest in the family slightly increased after having my suspicions aroused by my practitioner friend. Then indeed did I notice indications that both she and her husband lived very separate lives. To the outside world they might have seemed a close couple, but having been alerted I was able to detect signs of a relationship which displayed a tolerance towards each other to go their own ways, and pursue their own interests. They had obviously come to terms with a less than ideal relationship, but continued to live together for the sake of the children.

Having found that she could talk freely with my more experienced and mature colleague, this lady accepted his advice as to how to cope with the situation and this exchange helped her tremendously. He had managed to gain her confidence and she opened up, which made for an understanding relationship between patient and practitioner. She would always refer to him with great respect and fully realised how much he had helped her through these difficult times.

She eventually overcame her problems with the further help of some homoeopathic remedies; in those days the choice would have fallen on any of the following:

—*Natrium muriaticum;*
—Belladonna;
—a Valerian remedy.

Today, in such cases, I personally find that the Bach flower remedies can be of great help.

This case shows that if the migraine had been treated conventionally, ie with drugs, no success would have been achieved because drugs may have alleviated the symptoms, but the cause would have remained undetected. Indeed, it is likely that the frustration would have increased and the situation might have grown steadily worse.

On the other hand, I remember a young man who had been treated as a psychosomatic migraine patient. When I studied his case, I suspected that he had been wrongly diagnosed. He was an extremely complex character and at every discussion we had he would further confuse the issue by tabling new emotional problems. I could readily see why a diagnosis of psychosomatic migraine had been reached in the first place. He displayed symptoms which were characteristic of different kinds of migraines, to which could be added his emotional problems.

I decided to use the Dermatron machine — Dr Voll's infallible discovery — and hoped that this would enable me to find the true cause of his migraines.

I subsequently discovered that the trapezius muscle would swell up at certain times during the day and his neck would become very painful. Then a sickly feeling would follow, which eventually led to a migraine headache. It would have been easy to prescribe treatment of his neck problems at that point in time, but I had to find out why this swelling recurred so regularly.

What really intrigued me was that gases had built up in his stomach and he complained of biliousness. Often this was accompanied by diarrhoea and eventually the Dermatron test revealed that he had a peptic ulcer. After treatment for his ulcer, there was no further need for neck manipulation or for further treatment for his supposedly psychosomatic headaches, because they had disappeared in the process.

This was an excellent example of the theory that symptoms should not be treated alone, but that the causes have to be unearthed and treated. It also proves the point that only a correct diagnosis can result in a cure.

Strangely enough, migraines are more prevalent in women than in men; why this should be the case is a matter of some dispute among the medical profession.

Once I was asked to treat a seventeen-year-old girl. She told me that under certain circumstances she would first of all blush heavily, become very upset and nauseous and, finally, end up with a migraine. During our talk I realised that she was intensely shy and would carefully manoeuvre situations so that she could stay in the background. When she was required to meet people she would perspire heavily, blush to a bright red and that would signal the beginning of a migraine attack. The nausea would set in and she would become increasingly tense and be forced to withdraw from the company. This way, however, she would unwillingly draw attention to herself, which in turn caused further conflict and only made matters worse.

I decided that as a matter of priority she should be instructed in relaxation exercises, and I backed these up by some homoeopathic remedies. Although her condition did not improve overnight and we sometimes felt that we were engaged in an uphill struggle, in time she changed from an unhappy, insecure teenager into a happy and balanced woman.

These feelings of insecurity and oversensitivity which can rob people of every scrap of self-confidence have often been developing slowly since childhood. Pushy or domineering parents, or the experience of being teased excessively at school and made into a laughing-stock, can be the cause. This may well result in an inferiority complex of such dimensions, as in this girl's case, that medical help is necessary.

Many characteristics or influences can lead to psychosomatic migraines, such as jealousy, grief or dissatisfaction at work. Occasionally, migraines are used instinctively as an excuse, but mostly they are real enough and people will suffer physically because of an inferiority complex or other emotional problems.

I can tell you about another teenage girl who attended our clinic for a period of more than twelve months. This case will make you appreciate how strongly emotional imbalances can prevail. This girl suffered badly from migraines and her mother was at her wits' end. The girl withdrew more and more into her shell and although I had decided that she was clearly subject to psychosomatic migraines, I could not get through to her.

We just struggled on until, one day, out of the blue, her mother told me that her daughter had totally changed. As a nineteen-year-old now, her migraines had suddenly waned. She had got to know a sensitive and understanding young man with whom she was able to share her thoughts and inner fears. This had helped her to develop into a different person. He was the love of her life and I wondered if he realised that he unwittingly had cured her migraines.

Sentiments such as obsession, frustration or other neurotic conditions are quite often at the root of psychosomatic or emotional migraines. Generally it takes quite some time before these tendencies are unearthed and recognised and it is not till then that treatment can be commenced.

These days we are fortunate in that we have a choice of treatments which are suitable for such conditions. Among other techniques we can use are relaxation therapy, bio-feedback and autogenic training.

I also remember the lady who was convinced that her migraines were a result of a brain tumour. She had spent a large amount of money in her efforts to find a cure and would insist with whichever specialist she visited on having X-rays and brain scans. Every time she was again reassured that there was no indication whatsoever of a brain tumour, but she refused to believe this. Her migraines increased in intensity and frequency, which only made her more determined in her beliefs. Her balance was affected and this to her was a sure sign of a tumour.

As all previous investigations had shown nothing out of the ordinary, I realised that she needed gentle handling, because she was so highly strung. I decided to explain to her the principles of Kirlian photography and ask her to have some photographs taken.

Kirlian photography is a technique which enables us to show, in black and white, the flow of body energy. In 1939 the Russian engineer Semyon Kirlian was repairing an electro-therapy machine when he accidentally allowed his hand to move too close to a live electrode. As a result he received a shock, accompanied by a brilliant flash of light emitted by a spark of electricity. This aroused his curiosity and Kirlian wondered what would happen if he placed a sheet of light-sensitive material in the path of the spark.

He placed his hand behind the paper and repeated the process he had done involuntarily the first time round. When the film was developed, Kirlian saw strange, streamer-like emanations surrounding the image of his fingertips. He then discovered that each emanation had a different radiation pattern. He was now totally intrigued and devised further tests in order to capture the energy aura.

This principle has since been further developed and is now used successfully to find out if and where the energy flow is disturbed. This accidental discovery can also be applied to find accurate acupuncture points or "energy points", which can be used to block or stimulate energy or correct a disharmony in the energy flow, if so required.

In this lady's case a photograph of the aura of the brain would show indeed if there was an energy disturbance which could point to a possible brain tumour. The photographs came out beautifully and although the aura showed signs of great emotional stress, there was no indication of any serious irregularity.

I talked the whole process through with this lady with the

Kirlian photographs in front of us and began to notice a slight change in her attitude. I asked her if she was prepared to use some herbal and/or homoeopathic remedies and tried to instil in her some faith and trust that her problems could be overcome. Well, I am delighted to say that we did just that!

I concluded that homoeopathically she should be diagnosed as a Lachesis type of patient, as she had informed me of her difficulties in swallowing. She could barely swallow even liquids and she also had great difficulty in getting off to sleep.

When the impossible had been achieved (her own words), she said to me several times over: "Thank heaven that with your help I managed to crawl out of this self-created hell I have been living in."

In the present unfortunate climate of unemployment we come across examples of extreme anxiety when people have to go to the Employment Exchange, or for a job interview, knowing that there are dozens of others after the same job. As a result of their tension and anxiety they will end up with a migraine and realise they will not be at their best during the interview. If they do not get the position they were after, they will reason that it was due to the migraine. When the time comes for their next interview, the previous failure is still fresh in their memory and the process of anxiety resulting in a migraine will start all over again, ending in further disappointment.

These people would benefit greatly if they were to use any of the following homoeopathic or herbal remedies from Dr Vogel:

—Valerian
—Avena sativa
—Ginsavena

Sometimes also, aromatherapy or relaxation exercises will provide a solution. Relaxation therapy should include a low-stress diet, curtailing the intake of animal proteins.

A variety of situations can be the cause of individual psychological reactions resulting in a psychosomatic migraine attack. It is up to the doctor or practitioner to trace it back to its beginnings and not until then will it be possible to devise a suitable programme for treatment.

There is, however, no doubt that extreme stress and anxiety can lead to, among other things, physical and psychological suffering. If this results in migrainous attacks there is little point in feeling sorry for oneself and sitting back and letting it wash all over you. A positive attitude is needed to assist whichever doctor or practitioner is being consulted, in his or her efforts to affect a cure. If we run away from reality the practitioner will find it extremely difficult to help a patient with psychosomatic migraines, and the best advice I can possibly give is to stop running, turn around and face reality. I need hardly assure you that the effort will prove worth while in the end.

9

Ménière's Syndrome

ONE MAY BE surprised to see Ménière's Syndrome included in this book, which is largely concerned with migraines and, as such, Ménière's Syndrome seems to be a deviation from the subject. This assumption, however, is only partly correct as it is not unusual for a migraine sufferer to later develop Ménière's Syndrome.

It was a few years ago, while I was on a lecture tour of the United States, that a Scottish lady came to shake my hand after an evening lecture. She had attended our clinic in Scotland some twelve years previously, in connection with headaches and migraines which later developed into Ménière's Syndrome.

At that time I had treated her with acupuncture, together with several homoeopathic remedies, amongst them a German preparation called Dyscornut. I also had given her soft tissue palpation and manipulation and after all these years I was again able to witness the satisfactory results of that programme. At the time she had indeed been totally co-operative, because she was planning to emigrate with her

71

husband to the United States to be nearer her children who had settled there.

Ménière's Syndrome is one of those afflictions where feelings of giddiness can result from either a disease in the inner ear or a brain mechanism malfunction. In this lady's case there was considerable hearing loss due to a lesion in the inner ear and she also experienced neural hearing losses.

The existing migraine problem seemed to complicate things further. It had been a longstanding condition and she had not been able to find anyone who could advise her as to the correct treatment. Both she and her husband had reached desperation point as they wanted to emigrate and settle in the States before becoming too old for such an upheaval. Therefore I can assure you that it was a very happy couple who left us once her symptoms had completely disappeared after the treatment programme she followed.

Although Ménière's Syndrome patients often suffer a hearing loss, the opposite can also occur, which, in a way, can be an even worse handicap to live with and that is that they are intermittently plagued by sounds inside their heads. From my experience with patients I have treated for this condition, I would not consider it an exaggeration to describe this condition as an utterly debilitating existence.

I remember one occasion when I was walking back towards the clinic after a short lunch-break, when I saw a lady sitting in a parked car in the car park. By the time she entered the consulting-room I had already guessed what she had come to consult me about, because she had been sitting in the car, on her own, with earphones on. She told me that she would spend most of the day plugged in, on both ears, to a transistor radio in an attempt to drown out the noises inside her head.

After I had given this lady a thorough overall check-up I sent her first of all to our X-ray centre. Her own doctor, with whom she was very friendly, kindly supplied me with her case history and I came to the conclusion that she had suffered extensive damage to the auditory nerve. We came to know each other quite well and developed a mutual respect, for the simple reason that every time she returned for treatment she reported some measure of progress.

This may be considered a small wonder in cases of Ménière's Syndrome, because these patients react extremely slowly to any kind of treatment. I was dealing here with a tenacious lady, however, and she was determined she would see it through and recover, and indeed she did steadily improve. Occasionally she expressed her gratitude for the decrease in the noises which used to "drive her bonkers".

We have not managed to overcome the problem totally, but she can now live without having to be plugged into a transistor radio. She returns from time to time for a treatment session to keep this problem under control and recently I have been giving her some laser treatment, to which she is responding extremely well.

It does happen every now and then that a case which has been diagnosed as Ménière's Syndrome actually turns out to be of a more serious nature.

I remember a middle-aged gentleman who told me that he had been diagnosed as suffering from Ménière's Syndrome. I was not totally convinced of this when he described his progressive symptoms and insisted on a thorough examination by an ear, nose and throat specialist.

Afterwards I was glad that I had insisted on a second opinion, because it appeared that he had sustained some serious head injuries during an accident. After he had undergone brain surgery, his so-called Ménière's Syndrome symptoms disappeared and he became his usual self again without the need for further treatment.

Nevertheless, if we are dealing with a true case of Ménière's Syndrome, how do we set about tackling it? Usually, by the time patients end up on my doorstep they have exhausted the channels of orthodox treatment. "Nothing ventured, nothing gained" unfortunately seems to be the attitude most people take to alternative medicine. Mostly, however, I am able to help these people with the use of acupuncture, laser treatment, soft tissue palpation or manipulation. Some people will respond very well to this treatment, while others will report only a limited degree of improvement.

I have found that all Ménière's Syndrome patients benefit from Vitamin B3 or Niacin. The latter is also known under the names of nicotinic acid, niacinamide and nicotinamide and is a member of the Vitamin B complex group. In its capacity as a co-enzyme, Niacin assists enzymes in the breakdown and utilisation of proteins, fats and carbohydrates. Niacin is also effective in improving circulation and reducing the cholesterol level in the blood. It is vital to the proper activity of the nervous system and for formation and maintenance of digestive-system tissues.

Relatively small amounts of Niacin are present in most foods. Niacin is remarkably resistant to heat, light, air, acids and alkalines, but it is quickly lost in cooking. Niacin's precursor is Tryptophan, an amino acid that can be converted into Niacin by the body. Lean meats, poultry, fish and peanuts are rich daily sources of both Niacin and Tryptophan, as are such dietary supplements as brewer's yeast, wheatgerm and desiccated liver. Niacin may prove beneficial for problems such as Bell's Palsy, Ménière's Syndrome, tinnitus, high-tone deafness, headaches, migraines, Parkinson's Disease, vertigo and quite a few more.

My advice to Ménière's Syndrome patients is generally that they should start with a low dosage of Niacin, increasing it to possibly 100 mg daily; this is especially the case for the Ménière's Syndrome patient who also suffers from vertigo problems.

If migraines are also involved then additional doses of Niacin, ranging from 100 to 200 mg daily will help to relieve the acute migraine attacks. However, in these cases I would advise that the natural form of Niacin is used in preference to a synthetic form. In my experience it hardly matters what type of migraine we are dealing with; a high dosage of Niacin will always relieve the condition.

In some serious cases of Ménière's Syndrome I may choose to use the neural therapy from Dr Huenecke. I am also in favour of these patients doing some relaxation exercises and a variety of these can be found in my book on *Stress and Nervous Disorders*. I know only too well how much patients suffer from problems such as Ménière's Syndrome, and yet I also know how much can be achieved by maintaining a positive attitude.

I was taught a valuable lesson by a young house-painter. As the result of a fall from a ladder he had sustained some head injuries. Then it was thought that he suffered from Ménière's Syndrome. He had a positive mind and was determined to find help and in Dr Vogel's book, *The Nature Doctor*, he read about Arterioforce as a helpful remedy in cases of circulation problems. With his layman's understanding, he equated dizziness to circulatory problems.

He acquired a bottle of Arterioforce, which is a herbal composition of *Crataegus oxyacantha* (hawthorn berries and blossoms) and *Arnica montana*. Whatever became of the hospital diagnosis of Ménière's Syndrome, Arterioforce served him extremely well and left him a delightfully happy man, which goes to show just how much determination and a positive attitude can achieve.

The dizziness had not cleared totally, but after some minor osteopathic manipulation even that disappeared — and that was the end of his Ménière's Syndrome worries.

10

Tinnitus

AS I HAVE already explained in the chapter on Ménière's Syndrome, tinnitus also falls into that category of not actually being a migraine, but certainly closely related to one.

By now we have realised how wide a variety of migraines exists; this is also the case in conditions related to noises in the ear and/or head. Most of these conditions are grouped together under the name tinnitus.

The condition of tinnitus is variously described as hearing an intermittent or constant sound of ringing, buzzing, piercing, roaring or hissing. Its causes are manifold and I will mention some of these, but no importance should be attached to the order in which they are listed: infection, catarrh, meningitis, cardio-vascular problems, hypertension, arteriosclerosis, Ménière's Syndrome, allergic reactions, dental disorders, fungus problems, excessive smoking or drinking, over-use of drugs, and so on.

Whatever the cause of the condition, the symptoms are usually so bad that patients are prepared to go to any lengths to find treatment — like the doctor who travelled to see me from abroad to find out if there was anything I could possibly do to relieve him from this hell. The noises he heard were of such constant din that it was impossible for him to continue with his work, as his concentration was totally destroyed. When I told him that I only worked with alternative methods, he stressed that I had total freedom to use any method I thought necessary, as long as I could help him.

This was of course easier said than done, because tinnitus is not an easy problem to cure, and what is successful for one person may well be ineffective for the next. A different and individual approach is needed for each patient.

Another gentleman comes to mind who had recently returned from Indonesia, where he had been posted by his company. He had been working there under extreme pressure and had paid little attention to his diet. Atmospherical influences had taken their toll and he was suffering from an obstruction of the external auditory canal due to foreign bodies of an infectious origin, which had been treated in the Far East with heavy doses of antibiotics. I had to decide which homoeopathic remedies to use to eliminate from his blood the remnants of these infections and the antibiotics he had used — the miasmas.

He had initially suffered from trigeminal neuralgia, but the final outcome was a full-blown tinnitus. Sometimes with tinnitus we recognise a peripheral vascular problem and in this case the trigeminal neuralgia had affected various arteries and the resulting pain and noises were unbearable.

Neural therapy and acupuncture gave him only temporary relief, but by changing his dietary management we were able to rid him of the excessive toxicity. From the homoeopathic remedies suitable for this condition I chose Dyscornut, Echinaforce and Hyperisan. Both his problems were therefore treated and, when I occasionally meet him, I can see that the treatment was one hundred per cent successful.

Let me make it quite clear that I consider dietary management to be extremely important for any tinnitus patient. A good cleansing diet is essential in the general treatment programme for tinnitus and as such I would suggest that the liver diet is followed, which I described in the first chapter of this book.

I know that many more people than we may realise are occasionally hit by high-pitched ringing or buzzing noises in the ear. The pain can be cutting like a knife if certain noises are combined — and some people have been subjected to this for years. My advice to any chronic tinnitus patient is to use a high dose of Echinaforce, sometimes 30 or 40 drops, three times daily, in combination with Loranthus and Lachesis — the homoeopathic low-potency snake poison.

Although mechanical devices such as a tinnitus mask or a hearing aid may offer some relief, I still maintain that proper nutrition is half the solution. Here again, high doses of Niacin — 100 to 200 mg daily — will help to relieve the symptoms.

It could well be possible that tinnitus sufferers react adversely to certain foods. It is mostly with high-protein foods that allergic reactions are experienced. The allergic effects could actually increase the symptoms tenfold, and an understanding of this will lead towards appreciation of my insistence on dietary management.

When meeting a tinnitus patient for the first time, I will immediately make sure that they are aware of the dietary necessities and supplementary intake of vitamins, minerals and trace elements, after which I will decide on whichever therapeutic treatments would be considered suitable. I usually opt for acupuncture, because if there is pain involved, acupuncture will quickly ease those symptoms.

When I attended and lectured at a world conference of medicine recently, I met Dr Suleman Shaikh from Pakistan, who works as a consultant in the Department of Anaesthesiology in Karachi. The opportunity presented itself for a long talk and we discussed a variety of subjects. He told me about the many patients they treated for migraine, epilepsy and related disorders such as tinnitus. He believed that the tinnitus problem could be provoked by strong vasodilation, often producing headaches or increased noises in the ears. In all the different research tests his department had undertaken, his experience had been that drug therapy was of little use. In biochemical terms, however, much could be done for this condition and with acupuncture, working on the pituitary gland and the brain stem, substantial relief could be obtained.

I found it especially interesting that he used some traditional acupuncture points which I had learned about in China many years ago. He claimed a good success rate in the treatment of migraines and related disorders when using these little-known points.

Tinnitus is one of those conditions where alternative or complementary medicine may find an answer where orthodox medicine so far has failed. I therefore feel, with the hindsight of many years of experience, that no effort should be spared in order to procure a successful treatment for this drastic suffering.

I must stress again that a good dietary approach, with supplementary vitamins, minerals and trace elements, will contribute towards recovery from this affliction, which has succeeded in making life a misery for countless people.

11

Vertigo

THE LADY WHO was shown into my consulting-room grabbed me by the arm and, with a pathetic look on her face, she pleaded: "Please hold me or I'll fall."

If it had not been for that look of suffering people would be forgiven if they had assumed her to be drunk, as she was literally swaying on her feet. She looked pitiful. I knew immediately that she was suffering from vertigo. After helping her into a chair, I first of all listened to a summing-up of her symptoms in order to see whether I was dealing with a straightforward case of vertigo or if there was another factor involved. Like so many other conditions, a vertigo attack can also act as an alarm signal, pointing to a possible irregularity elsewhere in the body.

A true vertigo is perceived as a faint, dizziness or light-headedness. It is a disturbance of the equilibrium and can be due to an enormous variety of reasons. I will list some of these, in no particular order, but just as they come to mind: toxic conditions, middle-ear infections, obstructions, use of drugs, eyesight problems, blood disorders such as anaemia, leukaemia, infections or inflammations, haemorrhage, Ménière's Syndrome, epilepsy, migraine, cardio-vascular problems or hypertension.

By now you will be familiar with my viewpoint on treating the symptoms of a possibly far-reaching disorder, and you will understand that it could take quite some time to get to the root of the problem. Not until then will it be possible to decide on a course of action.

Osteopathic practitioners are in the happy position that their training has been directed towards bringing relief with manipulative treatment. They have learned what to look for, but although speedy symptomatic relief can be effected, they also know how imperative it is to find the cause of the problem. Any experienced practitioner will know how unwise it is to do any manipulation in the case of vertigo. Such an attack could well be an indication of a vascular problem such as high blood pressure or, even worse, of cardiac failure, and therefore great care is necessary in establishing a diagnosis before doing anything of the kind.

On the other hand, however, once the cause has been determined, the vertigo patient can be relieved of his or her symptoms almost miraculously with some relatively simple manipulative action. In this way the practitioner can easily restore the circulation of blood to the brain if the disruption was due to a lesion or a disc problem. Many vertigo sufferers have found quick relief when the circulation of the blood was restored with simple but careful manipulation. This must, however, always be done by an experienced professional, or else irreparable damage could be caused.

I remember feeling a certain hesitation when asked to treat a teenage girl. She would suffer irregular but violent attacks of vertigo, with no pattern whatsoever. Brain scans had not shown any sign of a physical irregularity, neither had the X-rays on which I had insisted. Her attacks would last from half a minute to a few minutes and would be accompanied by nausea and sometimes even vomiting.

It finally came about that a certain neck movement brought

81

on an attack and, indeed, I found an irregularity there on further examination. In this case, one session of manipulative neck treatment was sufficient to cure her of her vertigo attacks. Her general practitioner told me later that when she visited him, she had proudly said that a "bit of massage and a crack" had been the answer to the problems she had suffered for a few years.

Then there was the family where both parents were patients at our clinic. The mother told me of her shock when her son had come home and told her of his latest hobby, namely deep sea diving. She was not keen on the idea at all, but he had made up his mind. It was not long afterwards that she told me about these funny turns he had and I guessed that these were occasional vertigo attacks. I told her to ask him to come and see me and explained that divers are sometimes affected this way, probably as a result of the water pressure when their technique is not quite correct. After examination, I realised that indeed there were no other indications and I advised him to temporarily stop diving. I also gave him some tips which would prevent a recurrence of these problems when he eventually resumed his training.

It is not unusual for migraine sufferers to be affected by vertigo, either at the outset of an attack or afterwards. However, help is at hand in the form of Loranthus. The homoeopathic remedy Viscasan is also useful for such conditions and I will take this opportunity to point out how important detoxification is for vertigo patients. For this, I recommend garlic, extract of cereal grasses and beetroot juice. For the best results fresh beetroot should be used.

With the current increase in post-viral syndromes and especially myalgic encephalomyelitis, we see patients suffering dizziness and failure of motor function, ie problems with walking, the use of arms, failure of sensory regulation, headaches, failure of autonomic mechanism displayed in sweating, and several other comparable discomforts. The myalgic encephalomyelitis patient who is affected by dizziness or vertigo will always experience an improvement on a strict detoxification programme. For this I again find the liver diet excellent, together with Harpagophytum and liberal doses of Oil of Evening Primrose. Patients often claim that this basic treatment has ended their dizziness or vertigo discomforts.

The extract of couch grass — *Triticum repens* — is also beneficial for these conditions and its use has been described in detail in my book on *Traditional Home and Herbal Remedies* under the chapter on 'Roots'.

In alternative medicine we have access to a large assortment of remedies which have proven to be beneficial and I have many letters from patients who have written to express their gratitude and surprise that they had been cured with the help of remedies which they did not know existed. A London doctor, for example, whom I treated successfully for vertigo, used to monitor his condition with great interest and he has since developed a healthy curiosity in natural medicine.

Finally in this chapter we should consider the chronic vertigo patient with no other indications than circulatory problems or hardening of the arteries. Especially when these patients belong to the middle-aged or older generation, I would strongly recommend oral chelation therapy.

This is a fairly modern method. The tablets contain vitamins, minerals, trace elements and glandular supplementation, and, in short, it is a broad-spectrum formula which can be used without any danger of side-effects. We have experienced an entirely enthusiastic response to this therapy especially from the older generation of patients suffering from vertigo.

12

Convulsions

CONVULSIONS CAN DEFINITELY serve as a warning signal of a physical disorder elsewhere. Convulsions are violent involuntary contractions of the voluntary muscles, which sometimes repeat themselves. They could also be explained as spasms of muscular contraction interlaced with periods of relaxation, due to a disturbance of cerebral functions.

Of the several different types of convulsions, there are two major categories:

—the continuous contraction which is a cause of rigidity;
—the clonic contractions or a series of spasms alternating with periods of relaxation.

There are many factors which cause the body to convulse: infections, hypoglycaemia, cerebral oedema, a lesion in the brain, epilepsy, hysteria, tetanus, to name but a few.

How carefully these seizures must be investigated! I realised this again some time ago when a lady attended our clinic with her daughter. The mother told me that the girl had experienced one seizure after another. When I examined the girl I suspected that she was hyperventilating, thus causing the convulsions. I advised that her own general practitioner be consulted and he indeed confirmed my diagosis of hyper-ventilation.

As the range of possible reasons is so large, it goes without saying that the treatment ought to be adapted to suit each single person and that individual care and attention is necessary in each case. Having said this, the treatment for a person who is actually experiencing a convulsion or a seizure is fairly standard.

The first rule is never to panic. React calmly and take a folded tissue or handkerchief and place this between the teeth, taking care not to get the fingers trapped. Always unfasten collars or ease any clothing at the neck, so that the breathing is facilitated as much as possible. Place a pillow under the head and make the patient as comfortable as possible, preferably laid out on the floor. It is sometimes advisable to put a cold cloth over the top of the head, especially if the person concerned is an alcoholic.

Infantile spasms should be handled similarly. Make the child comfortable, watch it carefully, but do not panic. Above all, make sure that the person undergoing the seizure cannot injure himself by hitting or thrashing into hard or sharp objects.

Convulsive seizures are always the result of an acute disturbance of the cerebral function. We know that homoeo-pathic remedies exist for individual cases, and many people will gratefully testify to this fact.

There is a real possibility of a hereditary factor; if one or both of the parents are prone to convulsive seizures, this trend could also occur in their children. Especially helpful in those cases is Chickweed or *Stallaria media*. Although a common remedy, as a herbal treatment for convulsions, I regard Chickweed to be very beneficial and it certainly has proved successful in many cases. We know that convulsions may occur as part of the withdrawal symptoms after chronic use of drugs, alcohol or any addictive preparation or substance. Chickweed is a sure way to ease these withdrawal symptoms.

With cases of epilepsy it is said that by far the largest majority of the seizures are caused by the *grand mal* seizure, while approximately 25 per cent are from *petit mal* attacks. Psycho-motor attacks account for 18 per cent, displaying different combinations. Seemingly innocent fits of fainting should never be ignored, whatever shape or form they might take. If fainting occurs occasionally, one would be wise to have these occurrences looked into, to make sure that they are not the onset of a convulsive pattern.

If the seizures are diagnosed as being of a hypoglycaemic origin, take liberal quantities of Oil of Evening Primrose capsules. This is also very much advised for that small percentage of multiple sclerosis patients who may be prone to convulsions, and for diabetic or pellagra patients. All these patients will benefit from regular high doses of Oil of Evening Primrose.

I remember a patient who would experience only one convulsion a year. This had been occurring for a number of years and then it was found that the cause was an early skiing accident. After this accident the lady had suffered a convulsion, and every year around the time of the accident she would take another convulsion. I treated her with the Rescue Remedy from the range of Bach flower remedies, and backed up the treatment with Loranthus and Oil of Evening Primrose. This finally broke the unusual pattern of her convulsions.

We also find that metabolic therapy might be of help with convulsive patients. In many cases improvement follows when large quantities of Vitamin D are taken. Vitamin B6 has also proved beneficial for people who suffer fits or seizures.

The minerals magnesium and calcium may also have a remedial effect. I remember a young child who suddenly started with seizures and she was completely cured with the use of Vitamin B6 and Urticalcin, a homoeopathic siliceous calcium preparation. The mineral Dolomite may also be used for these conditions.

Let me also point out in this chapter that if there is a serious allergy problem, whether the patient be young or old, convulsions or seizures could result. It is most important that the substance to which the patient is allergic is detected. Do not forget that an allergy can develop at any age and just because there have been no previous signs of allergic reactions, this does not necessarily mean that the situation will remain unchanged.

I will also use this opportunity to issue an earnest warning that, with any kind of convulsion or fit, care must be taken with food additives. All food additives should be avoided or reduced as much as possible, as there may well be a connection. Likewise, coffee, tea, nicotine and alcohol should be considered out of bounds for anyone who suffers convulsive problems.

I remember a young girl who would experience a convulsion perhaps once every three months. Her parents were worried that this pattern could perhaps establish itself as an epileptic condition. I was doubtful because there seemed to be no reason why it should progress as there were no other indications. Even so, I still had to find the underlying cause of her seizures.

After having put this girl through several tests without finding any indications, I decided to carry out some allergy tests. It was then that I found the girl to be allergic to aluminium, and it transpired that her mother's cooking utensils consisted largely of aluminium. It was most likely that the girl built up towards an allergic reaction over a period of time and in her case this reaction displayed itself as a convulsive fit. The convulsions had a somewhat peculiar pattern. Her fits would start with heart-rending screams and she would appear to be suffering extreme physical pain. Then she would become physically ill.

This latter aspect of her convulsions was cured by Nux Vomica. The treatment as a whole included an antidote to aluminium, Loranthus and Vitamin B6 and her fits became a memory of some frightful experience in the past.

As this case illustrates, careful detective work may be

required to get to the root of the problem and when that is solved, both patient and practitioner can justifiably be satisfied.

Finally, I would point out that it is fundamental for anyone who is prone to seizures or convulsions to learn to relax and to that end relaxation exercises are very important. To this effect much can be done with one's hands.

To be fair, when a person witnesses a seizure or a convulsion for the first time, it is fully understandable that they become extremely disconcerted. However, remain calm and try to remember the general guidelines which I have outlined earlier in this chapter.

If someone close to you is subject to these conditions, try to effect relaxation by placing the palm of the left hand over the fourth dorsal vertebra, then place the right hand on top of that and supply gentle pressure. This will help to relax the convulsive person. The area of the fourth dorsal vertebra could also be palpated with the thumb of the right hand, which will produce a similarly relaxing effect.

Equally useful under these circumstances is to put the left hand over the navel, the right hand on top of the left hand, and to do the Hara breathing exercise which I have described in my book on *Stress and Nervous Disorders*.

Always remember:

All healing takes place under total relaxation.

13

Epilepsy

FOR MANY YEARS I helplessly followed the progress of deterioration of a very good friend of mine. Our friendship dated back to our school years together. At some time during his teens he unfortunately fell from a cart laden with bales of hay and suffered a nasty head injury. He seemed to have recovered well at the time, but after a while he admitted to occasional absent moments, which were then diagnosed as *petit mals*. These gradually developed into quite severe epileptic fits. Out of necessity, the drugs prescribed to him became stronger and stronger to try and contain this condition, but finally these themselves started to affect his general health in a detrimental manner.

I was forced to watch this deterioration from close by and I felt so very sorry for my friend, but at that particular time there was nothing I could do for him. It left me, however, with a lasting impression of impotence and if only I had known then what I know now I might have been able to help him to a certain extent. Unfortunately, by the time I learnt more about this affliction, it was too late.

Nowadays, I regularly see epileptic patients in the clinic and I can only be grateful that our knowledge on this subject has increased, and that complementary medicine enables us to help these people. Sometimes it has been possible to achieve a reduction in their intake of drugs, but there have also been many cases where we have managed to totally end their dependence on drugs.

The results of treatment depend largely on the condition of the patient and on his or her general health. Their mental attitude and a willingness to accept alternative help is also a very important factor.

Let us start, however, by first taking a closer look at what epilepsy actually is and at some of the ways these people can benefit from alternative treatment methods.

Merck's Manual gives a very good definition of epilepsy. There it is stated that epilepsy concerns a chronic paroxysmal disorder of cerebral function, characterised by recurrent attacks involving changes in the state of consciousness — sudden in onset and of brief duration. The attacks, which mostly resemble a convulsion, can be divided into the following three categories, each of which exhibits a specific pattern:

—the *petit mal*;
—the *grand mal*;
—the physical equivalent of psycho-motor attacks.

Epilepsy, as a medical condition, can be separated into two categories, namely idiopathic and symptomatic.

With idiopathic epilepsy, there is no sign of an organic lesion in the brain or any physiological disturbance which could point to a possible cause of the seizures. The majority of epileptic conditions fall into this first category.

With symptomatic epilepsy, however, an organic lesion in the brain or a physiological disturbance could indeed be the underlying basis of this condition. These lesions I refer to can range from tumours, degenerative problems, scar tissue or abscesses to traumatic or vascular injuries. Indeed, the cause of a seizure can be manifold.

Physiological disturbances again could be the result of many influences, such as alcohol, overdoses of drugs or insulin, hypoglycaemia, thyroid dysfunction, intracranial problems, whooping cough or cerebral oedema. Although there is no direct evidence that epilepsy is hereditary, certain disturbances may be present at birth which could be the cause of epileptic problems at a later stage.

It is always important, whether suffering from idiopathic or symptomatic epilepsy, that a programme is decided on for treatment and every effort should be made to find out as much as possible about which epileptic condition we are dealing with. It will aid the practitioner greatly if the patient is able to supply as much information about his or her family's medical history as is available. Then certain tests can be carried out and the results of these, together with the available background information, will hopefully enable the practitioner to reach the correct diagnosis.

Epileptic seizures are sometimes confused with hysteria, anxiety attacks, bouts of migraine, hypoglycaemic problems, narcolepsy or hyperactivity, as well as other problems which very likely are unrelated to epilepsy.

When a *grand mal* situation occurs, family or friends who are familiar with the behaviour pattern of the person concerned can quite often recognise the symptoms and may be prepared for what is happening. The patient will usually undergo convulsive tremors and spasms, lose consciousness and fall to the ground. Frequently this is accompanied by an initial scream, uncharacteristic sweating, excessive salivation and possibly tongue-biting and incontinence. The attack can last from two up to five minutes and when the patient regains consciousness, he or she may feel drowsy or confused and be left with a headache. These *grand mal* situations are of course most difficult to treat and yet even here it is possible that a well-balanced diet may greatly reduce the incidence of such occurrences.

The *petit mal* attacks are more common in childhood and willl last up to half a minute. However, these seizures can occur several times a day and care is obviously equally important.

Psycho-motor attacks differ from both the above-mentioned descriptions. Often these can best be described as a disturbance of consciousness without convulsions and a period of absence or amnesia can last from a few minutes to several hours, during which the patient behaves strangely and can possibly turn aggressive or violent.

You may now realise how important it is to take account of and eliminate any possible causative factors. The direct cause may be unknown, but by studying the combined factors a correct diagnosis may be reached. Once treatment has been established and the patient has been made aware of the situation, as normal a life as possible should be led.

No matter what the actual cause of the epileptic condition, it is of primary importance that any treatment method be based on a nutritionally balanced diet. An initial cleansing diet is therefore necessary to bring about a regular bowel action. Swimming, walking, cycling or any other physical exercising are recommended and, within reason, more extensive exercises should be encouraged.

As a result of long-term drug treatment, some unpleasant side-effects could eventually come to light and most doctors and specialists react favourably when asked to assist in reducing the patient's drug intake.

Minimal drug intake is of course most desirable, as with good dietary management, homoeopathic medication, herbal remedies and acupuncture, the frequency of seizures may be reduced considerably. In some cases the necessity for drugs has been totally eliminated under this treatment regime.

When treating an epileptic patient I will always endeavour to work closely with the doctor or specialist under whose care the patient originally was and who therefore knows the patient inside out as a result of tests and investigations done at his or her instigation.

My immediate and instinctive advice to any epileptic patient is to stress the importance of a well-balanced, nutritional diet, as I have witnessed substantial benefits from this in many of my patients. The outlines of the diet I advise for the control of epilepsy — both *grand mal* and *petit mal* attacks — are as follows:

Breakfast:
Half a grapefruit or a glass of unsweetened grapefruit juice.
Muesli, mixed with cooked prunes and prune juice or a handful of raisins and one apple and half a banana, chopped.
Porridge or bran.
Rye bread, brown rice or rye crispbread.

Lunch:
Salad using any raw vegetables, except tomatoes or cucumber. Alfalfa seed sprouts are especially recommended. Do not use too much cabbage.
Vegetable soup.
Rye bread, pumpernickel or rye crispbread.
Unsweetened natural yoghurt, or goat's milk or sheep's milk yoghurt.
Whole grains such as rice, barley or millet.
Boiled potatoes or jacket potatoes.

Dinner:
Lamb, game or poultry — no more than twice a week.
Trout or non-oily fish — no more than twice a week.
Pulses such as soya beans, aduki, kidney or haricot beans — at least twice a week.
Cooked fresh vegetables, including bean sprouts.
Brown rice and/or barley, millet and potatoes.
Non-sweet fruit such as grapefruit, rhubarb, apples, black-currants, gooseberries, blackberries.

Beverages:
China tea, Earl Grey or herbal tea, without sugar. Small amounts of milk can be used in India tea, but no more than one cup per day.

Elderflower tea, peppermint tea with a sprinkling of hops, or lemon balm tea.
Bottled spring water.
Grapefruit juice.
No sweetened fruit juices are allowed and where milk is used I would prefer to see soya milk used instead.

Dressings, oils and condiments:
Dress salads with lemon juice, or olive oil mixed with lemon juice or cider vinegar.
Use only sunflower or olive oil.
Use Herbamare or Trocomare salt or soya sauce.

Foods to avoid:
Sugar and sweet foods, foods cooked using flour and sugar, marmalade, chocolate, cheese, pork in any shape or form, oranges, tomatoes, peppers, sea fish, cucumbers, vinegar, common salt, red wine, excessive alcohol, sherry, port, instant coffee, processed and convenience foods, sweet fruits, sweetened fruit juices.

Supplements:
Take daily for a period from three to six months:
—50 mg Vitamin B6
—1 Stress B-Vite tablet
—500-1,000 mg Vitamin C
—500 IU Vitamin E
—2 Kelpasan tablets, first thing in the morning with a glass of warm water.

In order to obtain a good yin and yang balance in the diet, I suggest that brown rice features regularly on the menu. This should be carefully prepared according to the method which I have described in the first chapter of this book. This will ensure that the maximum nutritional value is maintained.

Over the years quite a few patients of mine have followed this dietary advice and, combined with other hints and remedies, their epileptic condition as well as their general health has improved greatly.

I remember a 42-year-old lady who told me at her first visit that she had been taking Epilim for many years. At first she had suffered from *petit mal* attacks, which finally resulted in several *grand mal* attacks. My programme for her consisted of the following:

—dietary changes;
—Loranthus, the Vogel herbal remedy based on mistle-
    toe grown on the wild oak;
—two tablets of Kelpasan taken first thing in the morning
    with some warm water;
—Vitamin B6

The results were extremely encouraging and since then she has been able to omit Epilim from her treatment altogether.

Then there was another female patient, still quite young, but she had been on the drug Epanutin for quite some time. Despite her condition she had given birth to a baby daughter by Caesarean section. Although she regularly suffered seizures before the birth, these completely disappeared afterwards. Instead she ended up with nasty migraines. I therefore treated her as previously described for migraines. Fortunately, the migraines disappeared and the young mother was completely cured. As a result she too has been able to eliminate the Epanutin treatment altogether.

I have already said that epilepsy cases often differ and, unfortunately, we are not always successful in our treatment. I well remember a young man who desperately wanted to be cured of his epileptic seizures. He had already been treated by several of my colleagues, and one of my best friends, a doctor with a great deal of experience, thought that his epilepsy could have been the result of a severe case of measles. This possibility had accidentally emerged during a conversation with the patient's mother. My friend therefore set out to attempt to remove the miasma left over from the measles with a homoeopathic Rubella formula. The initial reaction was tremendous and the young man improved greatly. However, several months later he again deteriorated and he then came to me. Whatever I tried, he still got worse and I was not even able to induce another remission let alone a lasting improvement.

Until this day we have not been able to reach any measure of success in this case. He has become mentally very involved in his problems and by now has adopted a negative attitude. As a consequence any positive advice we may give is now looked at with a great deal of scepticism. Neither with orthodox treatment nor with alternative therapies have we been able to help this unfortunate person.

Sometimes I wonder if atmospheric influences could have any bearing on epileptic persons. I have treated some of the worst *grand mal* cases, yet when they go abroad for a holiday quite a few of them have reported that they have had no attacks at all, while at home they would experience a regular pattern of one or two attacks a week.

There is the case, for example, of a young gentleman who is a patient at our clinic where we have been able to reduce the incidence of epileptic attacks considerably. He tells me, however, that when he goes to the Far East for his annual holiday, he never suffers any attack whatsoever.

Another memorable case is that of the young girl who suffered one or two *grand mal* seizures per week. She was completely cured of her attacks after acupuncture treatment with one needle at a certain point. She required no special diet or medication to supplement this treatment. I learned this technique from Professor Jayasurya when I worked with him at the General Hospital in Colombo, Sri Lanka. As Professor Jayasurya has been called on to treat many epileptics and nearly always uses this technique, I too have adopted this method.

Epileptic people tend to be rather nervous and then I advise them to take Loranthus and Valeriana each day. If they have a tendency to multiple fits daily, I recommend increased dosages of these remedies.

Hydrotherapy can also be of help and here a simple method is to direct a cold shower onto the back of the neck. This can be done equally effectively with a hand-held shower attachment above the bath.

Let us not forget, also, how important it is that epileptic persons take plenty of fresh air and exercise. In addition, the diet should contain plenty of raw vegetables, keeping meat consumption to a minimum.

Let me give you another example of how important a correct diagnosis is. I came across the worrying case of a young man who was extremely scared of doctors. Nevertheless, someone had tried to convince him that his problems could be epileptic seizures and he had finally succumbed and came to ask my advice.

In no way could I discover an epileptic aura and the symptoms to me did not relate to either a *petit mal* or *grand mal*. I persuaded him to see his own general practitioner in order to have certain tests done and was then informed that I had been right in my diagnosis. His problem was a relatively straight-forward migraine condition and here we were able to help him. The years of suffering and agony, also by his family on his behalf, had been totally unnecessary.

On the same subject, I should tell you about the lady who reported frequent epileptic seizures. She described the experience as being more or less in a vacuum and her mind going totally blank. Admittedly, her attacks sounded severe, but further investigation pointed strongly to hysteria. This condition caused problems which she then interpreted as epileptic fits. It was, however, due to something which took place only in her mind and her suffering was totally unnecessary. With guidance and mental training exercises, we were fortunate to be able to reverse the process, and she is now a great believer of the motto: "Mind over matter".

Allergic reactions can also resemble the symptoms of migraines or epilepsy. Some allergic people have been labelled as epileptics while in fact their attacks should have been ascribed to allergic reactions to certain foods. Controlled trials are necessary for such patients, as this not only happens with migraine sufferers but also with epileptic patients. The specific allergic reaction has to be determined in order to be able to treat these people.

These and similar cases are sometimes referred to as the "borderlands". The symptoms border on sleep, hysteria, delirium, or other conditions and are based on a neural level.

Although no exact cause of epilepsy is known, there is a possibility of an inherent factor in some cases. We do know that excessive use of alcohol can have far-reaching effects and if parents or grandparents used to imbibe excessively, the possibility exists that brain damage may have been caused, which could have repercussions for the following generation.

In cases where a hereditary factor is suspected it is sensible to base the treatment on the naturopathic foundations in which dietary adaptation, hydrotherapy and physical exercises feature. Exercises to improve the circulation should be done outside in the fresh air so that plenty of oxygen can be inhaled. For this reason it is sometimes advisable to include the mineral Germanium in the treatment, especially in the more severe cases. This will induce more oxygen into the bloodsteam and many people have benefited from this course of action.

Very often I use *Loranthus europaeus* in an extracted solution. Dr Vogel tells us that in former times old country doctors and nature doctors always used to prescribe mistletoe as a medicinal plant, because of its anti-spasmodic effect. Pseudo-epilepsy cases improve immediately with the use of Loranthus and are mostly cured. In East Africa Loranthus is known as a cure for many conditions, even malaria. The Bantu tribesmen recommend it specifically for all forms of epilepsy. In my opinion it is indeed, as Dr Vogel puts it: "a reliable remedy for epileptic derangements".

Minerals are also very important for epileptic people and magnesium and calcium are certainly often prescribed.

A young lady came to ask my advice on behalf of her very best friend — her dog. She had been told that her loyal and faithful companion was suffering from epilepsy. Although the dog's treatment had included bromide among the various drugs prescribed, it really had not improved the situation at all. I looked the dog over and asked her some pertinent questions concerning the duration and severity of the problems. She told me that the dog had been experiencing seizures since shortly after birth.

The use of bromide among the various drugs had ruined the poor animal's digestion, so I advised that he be given the homoeopathic remedy Nux Vomica, which I followed up later with some Belladonna 30 and Loranthus. The way this dog reacted was remarkable and he was completely cured of his seizures. In fact, the dog's character underwent some changes during the treatment period, which I therefore rounded off with the homoeopathic remedy Lachesis.

It is worthwhile to know that single homoeopathic remedies are suitable for the treatment of characteristic problems in both humans and animals, to rectify certain conditions. I want to stress once more that digestive disturbances deserve our full attention, whether dealing with *petit mal* or *grand mal* seizures, because it is most likely that the frequency of the attacks will be lessened if the digestive system works correctly. A controlled fasting programme should therefore be adopted, to be followed by the diet as outlined earlier in this chapter.

It is also true that epileptics can react favourably to spinal manipulation, acupuncture and laser therapy. Drinking and smoking should be considered out-of-bounds at all times. If and when the condition improves, the long-term drugs can then be slowly reduced under the close supervision of the doctor or practitioner who prescribed these in the first place. It would always be unwise to abruptly stop the drugs to which a patient has become accustomed often over a long period of time. This weaning must be a gradual process and during this period supplementary treatment, taking the form of homoeopathic or herbal medication, will then prove its worth.

Another case comes to mind concerning a lady who had

travelled abroad and forgotten her medication. She was in quite a state and was therefore recommended to visit a homoeopathic practitioner. He asked her how often she would suffer a seizure and she found this difficult to answer. Sometimes she would not have a seizure for a few months, while at other times she might suffer a more-or-less regular weekly attack.

She was then advised to take Vitamin D together with Dr Vogel's Kelpasan and to see how things went. She was delighted to tell me afterwards that during her holiday she had not had any fits and even on returning home nothing untoward had happened.

In cases of hystero epilepsy, which is a form of epilepsy connected with ovarium dysfunction, the fresh plant extract of mugwort is a very effective remedy. It is an excellent diuretic and encourages the menstrual flow. A few drops taken several times a day in a glass of water are recommended under those circumstances.

It is a known fact that immunological effects will alter the T-lymphocyte condition in times of stress. Therefore epileptic patients in those conditions should be especially careful with certain foods, such as sugar, meat, chocolate and spices. Some forms of relaxation like autogenic training or bio-feedback can be of help in such stressful conditions.

In conclusion on the subject of epilepsy, we have to say that according to a careful estimate there are over 300,000 epileptics in Britain today and each year a further 30-40,000 new cases are diagnosed. However, epilepsy is not a modern phenomenon; it seems to be one of the oldest diseases and writings exist dating back a thousand years or more which relate to this "sacred" disease. Fortunately, epilepsy is not a fatal disease, but on the other hand if it is not controlled it could shorten one's lifespan.

The central nervous system is composed of two different cells: the nerve cell or neuron, and the glia cell. These cells have different functions. The neuron transmits the nerve messages and activates various parts of the body and the glia is the soil into which the neurons are implanted. These need their support and they also need energy from food and, most particularly, a balanced energy between positive and negative.

All energy is vibration and all vibration is energy — and it all depends on what balance can be found. This is why the sciences of acupuncture and laser therapy are so essential in promoting a good balance between mind and body.

In quite a number of cases the cause of epilepsy remains unknown. Presumably it can be due to an inherent disposition or it may be the result of an infection, an injury, a tumour or any traumatic experience. Some patients find it disconcerting not knowing what the possible cause may be and perhaps, in their ignorance, they then encourage a thought process which may become a problem or even an obsession.

We should not overlook the fact that epilepsy is not a *disease* — it is a *symptom*. When looking for a possible single cause we have to bear in mind some of the physical or mental character-istics of the person involved. Only then can we aim to treat this particular affliction, not as a symptomatic disorder, but as affecting the whole of the person. Therefore a homoeopathic approach is particularly advantageous with epilepsy.

Traumatic experiences are quite a common cause of epilepsy. Figures are available which suggest that of approxi-mately 100,000 people admitted into hospital, about 5 per cent die of injuries, while a similar percentage develop epilepsy. Obviously, the sooner treatment is sought the less chance there is of the condition getting out of control.

Tumours or degenerative disorders, such as Alzheimer Disease, may encourage us into thinking that we are dealing with epileptic symptoms, as a gradual loss of neurons takes place. Our body contains billions of body cells, but we should nevertheless realise that with every tick of the clock thousands of them die. Therefore it is absolutely necessary that energy-building cell renewal should take place and to achieve this nutritional food is of prime importance.

In some cases it is possible to encourage the cell renewal

process with fresh-cell therapy, which can be given by injection.

The majority of epileptic patients seem to experience epileptic fits in their sleep, a smaller group do so while awake, and a minority belong to a combined category of the two. It is therefore wise to watch at which times the seizures take place and to see if there exists a pattern. It is also important that medical help is called for in the following instances:

- —if a seizure lasts longer than five minutes;
- —if the patient does not recover consciousness within fifteen minutes;
- —if the patient has injured him or herself during the seizure;
- —if a second seizure follows shortly after the previous one.

Any alternative methods available should be exhausted. Do not despair, but keep trying. I remember the young man who had become so despondent because of his condition that he had grown very moody. After he was persuaded to use some alternative remedies and treatment he felt more in control and more involved, and his moods changed for the better. He felt happier in himself and, possibly as a result of this, his fits became less frequent.

There is still much to be learned about epilepsy, but fortunately the future brings more and more enlightenment. We have come to understand more about body energies and also have come to appreciate the need for relaxation. Happily, epilepsy is no longer considered as a most horrific disease, but there is more understanding towards this problem. There are also many more methods available to us nowadays which can be applied in an attempt to control epilepsy, and even cure it.

The epileptic patient will benefit from a close co-operation between orthodox and alternative practitioners, where combined treatments could complement each other. This condition also requires a positive approach from the patient and his or her full commitment. Then it may be possible that with one treatment method or a combination of several therapies, a cure can be effected. Despite our acquired knowledge so far, we are still only able to scratch the surface of all that energy entails, but further research and an open mind will give us more insight and knowledge.

I was delighted to hear again from a young mother just a few weeks ago. She had come to bring me up to date about the condition of her three-year-old daughter who had suffered from *petit mal* seizures since shortly after birth. This child no longer needs to use any of the previously prescribed drugs and her fits are now very much under control. This was achieved with sensible treatment and the help of some homoeopathic remedies: Loranthus, Skullcap and Pimpernel.

Isn't nature wonderful, considering that it supplies us freely and in abundance with these remedies!

14

Practical Advice

TO ROUND OFF this book I would like to give some hints and advice which can be used to relieve the general discomfort migraine and epilepsy patients are intermittently subjected to. These simple guidelines have proven their worth with many patients in our clinic and if exercised correctly they will always stimulate the progress without interfering with the advised treatment programme. These advisory notes are for the benefit of anyone in these circumstances and should be regarded as being complementary to any recommended treatment.

Hydrotherapy — water treatment — is as old as mankind. Over many centuries people as well as animals have realised the value of water treatments. Water has been used not only for hygienic purposes, but also for its therapeutic value. The famous Greek physician Hippocrates, often referred to as the "Father of Medicine", put great store by water treatments and some of the Roman Caesars built as many as 170 bathing establishments between them.

These public bathing facilities were used extensively, not

only for the luxurious and hygienic qualities they offered, but because they were also considered to be beneficial to one's health. Much of the Roman citizen's social life was spent in the congenial and relaxing atmosphere of the public baths.

In Britain there were quite a number of spa towns which were used for their health-enhancing properties by the upper classes and landed gentry during the eighteenth and nineteenth centuries. It was then considered totally acceptable, in fact sometimes even as a social commitment, to take up temporary residence in a spa town for a few weeks every now and then to enjoy the waters. Of course, the most famous spa town in Britain was Bath, city of Avon, which was actually built by the Romans in AD 50 on the site of the thermal springs.

The mildest form of water treatment is the cold spray, which stimulates and improves the circulation. The whole of the body can be sprayed, or it could be restricted to certain parts of the body. This treatment is now within everyone's reach with the existence of modern-day showers, especially those with a moveable handspray. For migraine sufferers it is recommended to direct this spray onto the cervical vertebrae. Great relief can be experienced by doing this. Cold or semi-cold baths can be of help, as also can a bath at body temperature (37° Centigrade) when using a firm brush on selected parts of the body.

A partial steambath for the head can also be of help. The patient sits by the table in front of a bowl of steaming water to which a small quantity of Po-Ho oil has been added. This is an aromatic oil from the Vogel range of herbal products and contains the following plants:

—*Menthae piperita* (peppermint)
—Eucalyptus
—Juniper
—*Carum carvi* (caraway)
—*Foeniculum vulgare* (fennel)

Bend over the bowl and drape a towel over the back of the

head and allow this to reach the table so that the steam is trapped underneath the towel and can therefore be inhaled. This will relieve the breathing and the beneficial effects will be increased if afterwards a hot cup of chamomile tea is sipped. This simple treatment will provide a soothing effect for any kind of headache.

In the case of more severe headaches, however, or a migraine, I would advise that an ice-cold compress is placed on the forehead. Also the 'cold dip treatment' as outlined in Chapter 6 on hemiplegic or circulatory migraine, is a useful form of hydrotherapy.

The following saying has been ascribed to Priesznitz: "All that needs healing can be healed by water and the best pharmacy is water obtained from a fresh water spring." All his healing methods were based on any one or on a combination of hydrotherapy, diet, exercise, massage and fresh air.

Father Sebastian Kneipp, who also based many of his healing practices on water treatment, is famous for his statement: "Water may be used to calm, to stimulate, to eliminate and to influence the blood circulation." Certainly hydrotherapy, in whichever form it is used, will never clash with other forms of treatment.

I would now like to draw your attention to another method which can be used to ease those conditions dealt with in this book. Basically it is extremely simple, because I am referring to a fast. To fast successfully it is not just a matter of refusing to take any food whatsoever; you must take some liquids as they are absolutely necessary to avoid dehydration. A fasting period of one or two days will have a healing effect, as it encourages the elimination of toxins from the body.

Again, there is not much new under the sun, because in the Bible we often come across references to a fast. Philippus Paracelsus, a sixteenth-century Swiss physician, was also aware of the value of fasting and made mention of it several times in his medical works.

In our residential clinic we would always maintain one day of fasting each week. On that day at the usual times of breakfast, lunch, dinner and supper, our residential patients would be offered a choice of either mineral water or fruit juices. This method ensures export combined with the minimum of import, which inevitably causes any toxins to be released.

Every now and then I am asked questions regarding the safety of a course of fasting. Although it is possible to fast for a longer period of time than I have suggested, this must always be done under medical supervision. Please be sensible and do not attempt this without the knowledge and approval of your physician.

Sometimes it is good to take only fruit for a few days and then one can slowly start to reintroduce either water and/or fruit juices. Most herbal teas may be also used effectively during a fasting period. It is important that after a course of fasting, good dietary management be practised and the build-up is slow when solid food is reintroduced.

My general experience over the years has been that migraine patients benefit most from the liver diet (Chapter 1) with the inclusion of one day of fasting per week. Epileptic patients may also insert one day of fasting a week in their dietary management.

While on the subject of fasting I must clear up some basic misconceptions about this treatment. Some people believe that neither food nor drink should pass their lips during a fast and others reckon that fasting is all about no solids being allowed, but that any fluid or liquid is permitted. I must stress that the liquid intake may not include tea or coffee, as these products are toxic in themselves and are of no benefit to our health whatsoever.

I doubt if it is necessary to mention the fact that for obvious reasons any alcohol intake is also disallowed. We all know that alcohol can cause addiction problems, but possibly not everyone realises that the same goes for tea and coffee. Ask anyone who is used to drinking large amounts of either tea or coffee and they will tell you about their headaches when they suddenly, for whichever reason, drop that habit.

The reactions of some very severe migraine patients may, however, be different. I have sometimes been told that a measure of relief was obtained after they had drunk a cup of coffee. I find it even stranger when I hear that an alcoholic drink had brought relief. I do not really believe that either is true and suspect that this is more a psychological reaction, ie a bit of wishful thinking. I have seen too often that if and when these people were prepared to follow good dietary advice, they then reported real improvement. Although caffeine has been used occasionally as a medicine, this "medicine" has no place in a sensible naturopathic approach. I am sure that every person who is addicted to coffee will be in full agreement with this.

Coffee does not work as a tranquilliser or a relaxant, instead it is much more of a stimulant and can result in insomnia or feelings of unrest. Some people become aggressive after having drunk a lot of coffee or experience palpitations, although they are mostly unaware of the connection.

And what about all those people who suffer from ulcers? Certainly, as the liver and kidneys both play a major role in cases of migraine, they deserve a rest from coffee, tea or alcohol.

Epileptic patients, too, will not benefit from excessive amounts of coffee, tea or alcohol. A good herbal tea such as skullcap, vervain or mistletoe is of much more help to them.

The traditional naturopathic views of a well-balanced diet, plenty of water and fresh air being imperative to a healthy existence, still apply. The dietary advice given in this book is based on years of experience. Did Sir Robert McCarrison not say: "The greatest single factor in the acquisition and maintenance of good health is perfectly constituted food"?

I also want to give an earnest warning against smoking. It is not only with problems such as those discussed in this book, but under any circumstances, smoking should be considered a health hazard. I would therefore advise any smoker to try his or her utmost to break the habit.

I have already touched on the next subject several times,

but would like to enlarge on it here. That subject is relaxation. In addition to the specific breathing and relaxation exercises found in my book on *Stress and Nervous Disorders*, there are also other methods available such as bio-feedback, autogenic training and visualisation techniques.

I will explain an easy visualisation method which I have suggested many times to migraine and epileptic patients alike. Not only is it a useful method, but also relaxing and quite pleasant. All it needs is a little imagination and some concentration.

Make yourself comfortable in an easy chair with the head supported and the feet flat on the floor. Breathe in calmly and listen to the inhaling and exhaling. Take a deep breath and when expiring remind yourself to relax. Do this three times.

Now you are going to consciously relax all the muscles of your body. Begin with your eyes and mouth — squeeze the face tightly together and suddenly let go. Consciously relax the neck, shoulders, arms, hands, stomach, back, upper legs, calves, ankles and feet. In fact, try to relax every part individually and you will succeed in relaxing these parts.

When this has been done, try to remember a beautiful place where you have perhaps spent a holiday, or visualise a place which you would like to visit. It could be a beautiful lake somewhere, or a mountain range or an attractive coastal scene. Imagine yourself there and stay with that memory for a few minutes. This pleasant interlude is the introduction to the major part of the exercise.

Now you are going to look at your problem with your mind's eye, your head and your brain. You are going to see with your mind's eye how you yourself can help these problems and you visualise the blood vessels rushing in fresh supplies of blood, laden with vitamins and minerals. You imagine the building of new cells. As long as you try to see with your mind's eye how you can possibly help yourself to be complete, healthy and free from pain, you will reach this goal with a positive mind. You may use your own imagination, if only you see your problems abating and your defence system growing stronger and stronger. Once again you will be a healthy being.

Then the time has come to close the door on this mental picture and you breathe in and out consciously again three times, after which you may open your eyes. Then you may give yourself a pat on the back for having done so well.

Do this exercise programme three times a day, on waking, at lunchtime and on retiring. Withdraw to a quiet room and concentrate; empty your mind of everything else. Do not, however, force yourself; just build up a mental picture of the workings of your body. What you are in fact doing is comparable to reprogramming a computer. Although success is not likely to be immediate, rest assured that it will work.

Now I want to concentrate for a moment on the hands. Such a tremendous amount can be achieved with our hands that I could write a whole chapter about it. Few people are aware, however, of the energy which we possess in them. No fear, I promise that I will keep it short!

One simple exercise with the hands is to put the left hand on the occipital area — the bottom of the skull and the top of the neck — and the right hand on the forehead. Sit quietly in that position for a few minutes to relieve tension.

The Hara breathing method is also very good for general relaxation and this is found in detail in my book on *Stress and Nervous Disorders*.

Take relaxing holidays when possible, with some physical exercise and lots of walking in the fresh air. It is important not to break too much from routine and that mealtimes are not upset too often. Regular mealtimes are important because if the blood sugar level is allowed to drop too low, the risk of an epileptic fit or a migraine atttack increases. In this context I should again point out how much benefit may be obtained if Oil of Evening Primrose is taken regularly.

Now we come to the tissue salt remedies. These are quite safe to use and available for many different purposes, although I will only list below those which apply to the subjects of this book:

110

Calcarea Phos.	—for cold feelings in the head, soreness to touch, or for gastric problems.
Calcarea Sulph.	—for headaches with vertigo indications, nausea or a pain in the forehead.
Ferrum Phos.	—for general relief, for epileptic fits with rushes of blood to the head.
Kali Mur.	—especially when there is a sluggish liver, a furred tongue and sick headaches. Excellent general tissue remedy for epilepsy.
Kali Phos.	—for neuralgic headaches, menstrual headaches and especially if there is weariness and irritability. For epileptic persons who feel cold after a seizure.
Kali Sulph.	—for dull headaches.
Magnesia Phos.	—for convulsive habits.
Natrium Mur.	—sick headaches with diarrhoea.
Natrium Phos.	—for frontal or occipital headaches, especially on wakening in the morning.
Natrium Sulph.	—for colic pains.
Natrum Phos.	—useful for alternating a remedy and for intestinal problems.
Natrum Sulph.	—for traumatic epilepsy and head injuries resulting in spasms.
Silicea	—for nocturnal epileptic convulsions.

As we near the end of the chapter and the book I would like to summarise some of the general herbal remedies which

111

have proven so beneficial for migraine and epileptic patients.
These are as follows:

Avena sativa	—an extract of fresh oats — for insomnia, irritability and for strengthening of the nerves. A good breakfast of porridge will not do anyone any harm, but for those of especially nervous disposition *Avena sativa* is excellent.
Betula pendula	—an extract of the silver birch which serves as a diuretic.
Chelidonium majus	—extract of the celandine — more or less similar function as *Taraxacum*.
Lavendula officinalis	—lavender — of which the oil is used in two relatively new treatment methods, namely aromatherapy and reflexology (foot pressure). The lavender oil has a calming and soothing effect.
Loranthus	—an extract of mistletoe grown on the wild oak — for brain spasms and epilepsy.
Solidago virgaurea	—an extract of the Golden Rod — stimulates bladder function.
Valeriana officinalis	—an extract of the valerian plant — for neuralgia, headaches, cramps and fainting spells, stomach cramps and nervous anxieties.
Taraxacum officinalis	—an extract of the dandelion root — to ensure correct functioning of gall bladder, kidneys and liver.

Each and everyone of the remedies mentioned can be used singly. However, sometimes practitioners will recommend a combination and it is then we appreciate that there are still some herbalists who are able to combine mixtures to exact requirements.

To put it in a nutshell: never panic, but give nature a fair chance, because she is the ultimate healer. Do not throw in the towel if at first no improvement can be noticed. It could be that more time is needed or possibly that another remedy may be more suitable for your physical make-up.

I will take my leave with a quote from John Milton:

> Accuse not nature,
> She has done her part.
> Do thou but die.

Bibliography

Dr Willem Kremer — *Allergische Ziekten etc.* (4th edition, 1939), Van Hoekema en Warendorf NV, Amsterdam.

Dr John Mansfield — *The Migraine Revolution* (1st edition, 1986), Thorsons Publishing Group, Wellingborough, NY.

Ross Horne — *The Health Revolution*, Ross Horne, 21 Trappers Way, Avalon Beach, NSW, Australia.

Drs Boericke and Denvey — *The Twelve Tissue Remedies*, Boericke and Tafel, San Francisco, USA.

The Merck Manual (14th edition), Merck, Sharp and Dohme Ltd, Hoddesdon, Herts.

Oliver Sacks — *Migraine, Evolution of a Common Disorder*, Pan Books, London and Sydney.

Keith Mumby, MB ChH — *The Food Allergy Plan*, Unwin Paperbacks, London, Boston, Sydney.

P Heinsberg — *Natuurgeneeskunde in de praktijk*, La Riviere and Voorhoeve, Zwolle, The Netherlands.

Dr Alfred Vogel — *Nature, Your Guide to Healthy Living*, Verlag A Vogel, Teufen, Switzerland.

Peter Evans — *Mastering Your Migraine*, Granada, London, Toronto, Sydney and New York.

Harry Benjamin — *Everbody's Guide to Nature Cure*, Thorsons Publishers Int, Wellingborough, NY.

Dr A Vogel — *The Swiss Nature Doctor*, Verlag A Vogel, Teufen, Switzerland.
Lewith GT, MA, MRCP, MRCGP — *Alternative Therapies*, William Heineman Medical Books, London.
Peter Hazeldine — *Epilepsy*, Thorsons Publishing Group, Wellingborough, NY.

Other titles in the Series

Neck and Back Problems *The Spine and Related Disorders*	185158 084 0 cloth 185158 083 2 paper	£7.95 £3.95
Arthritis, Rheumatism and Psoriasis	185158 027 1 cloth 185158 028 X paper	£7.95 £3.95
Do Miracles Exist?	185158 029 8 cloth 185158 030 1 paper	£7.95 £3.95
Traditional Home and Herbal Remedies	185158 011 5 cloth 185158 012 3 paper	£7.95 £3.95
Multiple Sclerosis	0 906391 97 0 cloth 0 906391 98 9 paper	£7.95 £3.95
Stress and Nervous Disorders	0 906391 80 6 cloth 0 906391 81 4 paper	£7.95 £3.95

The above titles are available through all good bookshops and direct from Mainstream Publishing, 7 Albany Street, Edinburgh EH1 3UG.

NECK and BACK PROBLEMS
The Spine and Related Disorders

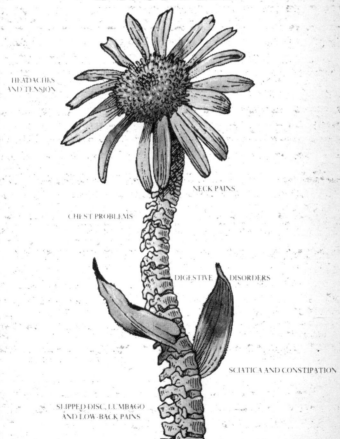

HEADACHES
AND TENSION

NECK PAINS

CHEST PROBLEMS

DIGESTIVE DISORDERS

SCIATICA AND CONSTIPATION

SLIPPED DISC, LUMBAGO
AND LOW-BACK PAINS

From the BY APPOINTMENT ONLY series

JAN DE VRIES

ARTHRITIS, RHEUMATISM AND PSORIASIS

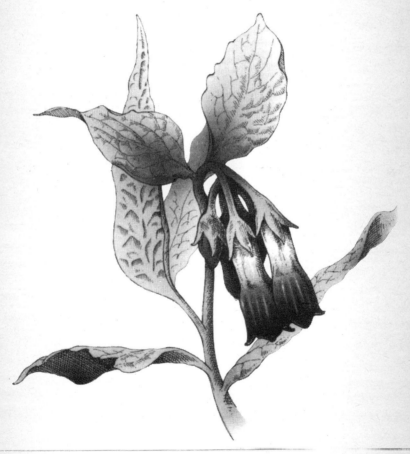

From the BY APPOINTMENT ONLY series

Winner of the Dag Hammarskjöld Award

DO MIRACLES EXIST?

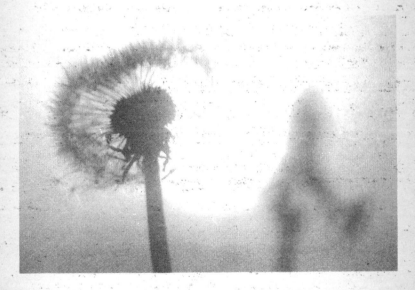

From the BY APPOINTMENT ONLY series

Introduction by Michael Van Straten

JAN DE VRIES

Traditional Home & Herbal Remedies

Introduction by Dr Alfred Vogel
Author of `The Nature Doctor´

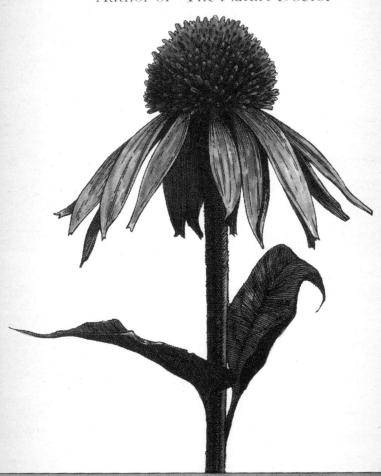

From the BY APPOINTMENT ONLY series

JAN DE VRIES

BY
APPOINTMENT
ONLY

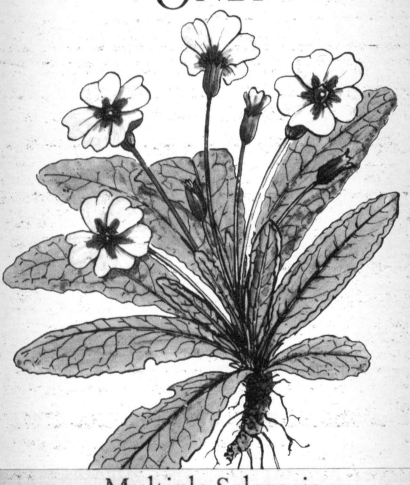

Multiple Sclerosis

Stress And
Nervous Disorders

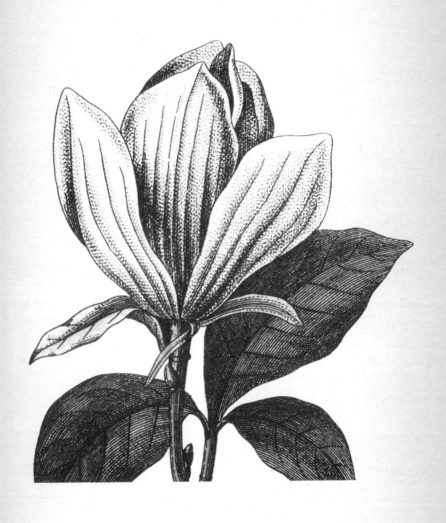